AGE
STRONGER

TO MY FAMILY, THE FUTURE, AND AGING STRONGER ACROSS GENERATIONS.

Quarto.com

© 2025 Quarto Publishing Group USA Inc.
Text © 2025 Mathew Wiest

First Published in 2025 by Fair Winds Press,
an imprint of The Quarto Group,
100 Cummings Center, Suite 265-D,
Beverly, MA 01915, USA.
T (978) 282-9590 F (978) 283-2742

Fair Winds Press titles are also available at
discount for retail, wholesale, promotional,
and bulk purchase. For details, contact
the Special Sales Manager by email at
specialsales@quarto.com or by mail at
The Quarto Group,
Attn: Special Sales Manager,
100 Cummings Center, Suite 265-D,
Beverly, MA 01915, USA.

29 28 27 26 25   1 2 3 4 5

ISBN: 978-0-7603-9350-5

Digital edition published in 2025
eISBN: 978-0-7603-9351-2

Library of Congress Cataloging-in-Publication
Data is available.

Design: Samantha J. Bednarek,
samanthabednarek.com
Photography: Herrington Health LLC

Printed in China

AGE STRONGER

PREVENT PAIN.
PRESERVE MOBILITY.
AGE RESILIENTLY.

Dr. Matt Wiest

FAIR WINDS

CONTENTS

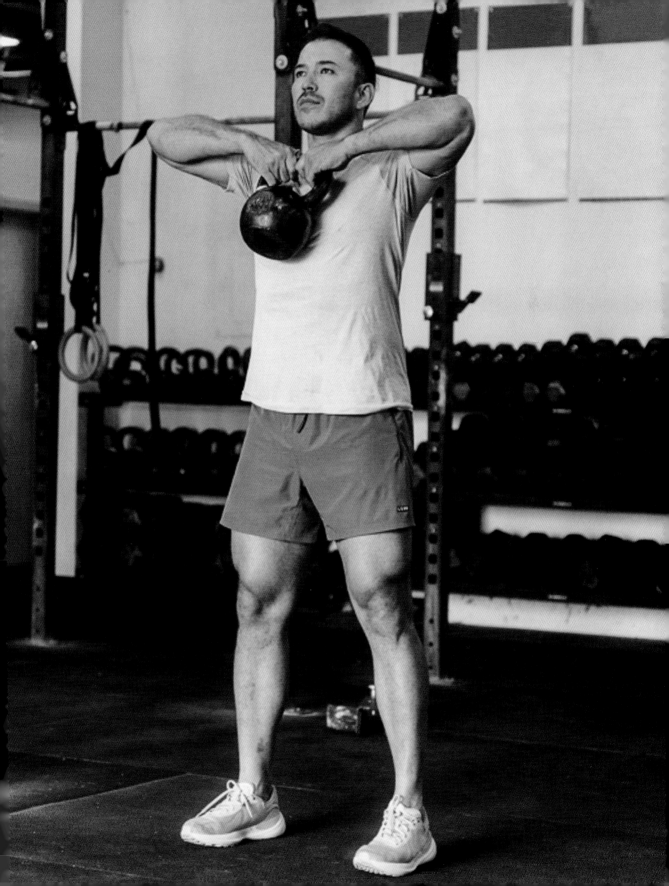

INTRODUCTION

Aging strong means recognizing our resiliency, leaning into the tools we have, navigating pain, and feeling confident about building strength.

Throughout life, though, we become conditioned to believe we are slowly falling apart. Our physical health is often compared to inanimate objects, such as appliances and cars. Terms like "wear and tear" and "blow out a joint" are almost the norm when discussing anatomy, aging, and the human body.

The reality is that the aging experience is more complex than these oversimplified ideas because we are not a rusted old F-150 with a slightly "off-center" axle (though some days may feel like it). We are dynamic, adaptable creatures who *crave* environments to thrive in.

Over the last decade, I have worked with thousands of people looking for hope and solutions to feel strong and age gracefully. I spent most of my early career years searching for tools and techniques to work *on* my patients. Recently, though, I have shifted my focus, spending less time on things like trying to discover the next best adjustment or quick-fix therapy, to investing more time working *with* patients by answering these questions:

- "How can I empower my patients to feel less fragile?"

- "Why does health care focus less on basics like stress, sleep, fuel, and movement in relation to pain management?"

- "Where can my patients find more support in community? Pain can be a lonely, shameful place. Is the current health care system improving or perpetuating it?"

- "What motivates people to make change, take ownership, and reclaim their health?"

- "How can people feel prepared for daily living, with confidence in their body's abilities as they age?"

ABOUT THIS BOOK

This book is structured with inspiration from Maslow's hierarchy of needs (typically depicted as a pyramid), but with regard to physical well-being and aging strong and with resilience.

Part 1 of this book—the base, or foundation, of "my" pyramid—is vital because it supports all other levels of the pyramid. The foundation comprises our "basic needs" of physical health, such as mindset, navigating stress, sleep, fuel, and social relationships and support—needs often neglected because society wants fast results, and focusing on these basic needs rarely yields quick change. I'll show you, however, that these critical areas affect our ability to build strength, and teach you strategies to build a support system, manage stress, and reverse limiting beliefs about your physical health. Meeting these foundational needs will allow you to move up the hierarchy and achieve higher levels of performance and well-being.

Part 2, next up on my pyramid, addresses full body, or "functional movements," a.k.a. daily living—carrying heavy groceries, sitting to standing, reaching overhead, or getting up off the ground unassisted. When thinking about these topics, we can get fixated on the *how* versus the *why*: How do I eliminate my knee pain? How do I get more mobile hips? How do I manage this lower back pain? Remembering *why* we want to feel strong and resilient can be overlooked in the process, and it's easy to become overwhelmed with advice and solutions that may not even apply to your body or need. Part 2 teaches you ways to scale full-body movements you need capacity for as you age.

I offer instructions on ways to build the necessary strength, mobility, balance, and control for activities that help you age strong and maintain independence, well-being, and self-esteem.

Part 3, at the top of the pyramid, explores specific areas of the body: feet, ankles, hips, core, neck, shoulders, and upper and lower back. The focus is on building strength and mobility, which can be a game changer for maintaining independence as you age . . . but only after establishing the foundation of the pyramid. Part 3 includes isolated exercises targeting things like shoulder strength and hip mobility that build on the exercises in part 2.

We live in a time with so much information available. This often results in half the population looking for a new way to "hack" health and the other half feeling overwhelmed. It is important to recognize that aging strong can look different for different people, so remind yourself not to get lost in the minutiae of every new, flashy health trend, and focus on consistently working on those basic needs to build the strong foundation you need to age strong.

My mission is to inspire people to reinvest in the basics, to feel empowered through movement, and to cultivate education and clarity around how to become their most resilient selves through all phases of life.

PART 1

Basic Needs

CHAPTER 1

REFRAMING SELF-TALK AND EXPANDING PHYSICAL CAPACITY

Understanding the power of self-talk—and the influence of the stories we tell ourselves about our body—is a critical component to building a foundation of well-being. The way we perceive pain, physical strength, and aging shapes our path forward. Of course, we face limitations out of our control, but we can shift how we view our physical health, which can create a positive trajectory toward aging strong.

The body narratives here are not from real people but are common things I have observed over the last decade in clinical practice. When people come to me for solutions, they *think* they want a new stretch, new routine, or the best treatment to reach their health, vitality, and fitness goals. The reality is that these things might help, but not without a solid foundation. Positive self-talk and how you perceive your capacity are fundamental parts of this and so powerful when building strength, recovering from pain, and aging with resilience.

I'M JUST GETTING OLD: BREAKING THE CYCLE

"I'm not even sure why I'm here" were Jim's first words. Jim, a recently retired fifty-eight-year-old, came to me hesitantly looking for help with recurring stiffness in his hips. After months of him complaining, his wife finally persuaded him to do something about it.

"We have a trip to the Appalachians next month and my wife is worried I won't be able to hike unless I stretch my hips—but I don't think there's much I can do. I'm just getting old."

I had him stand up and move around to get a general sense of how he was doing, but everything I asked him to do was met with minimal effort and interrupted by something along the lines of "Twenty years ago I could do this . . ." Jim had a tone in his voice I've heard many times. He was dismissive and set in his ways. He didn't have hope or room to believe much was possible outside of his current reality. His story was that he was caught in a cycle of chronic stiffness and discomfort that was a product of his aging body.

The more I got to know Jim, the more I realized his frustrations were rooted in the stories he was telling himself. He was convinced he was too old to make any changes; he was convinced that feeling the way he did was "normal" for someone his age; he was convinced this was the only reality that could exist for him.

Jim's is a common story. We (especially in Western civilizations) look for a "reason" or a direct cause of our issues that is out of our control, because then we cannot be responsible. This is easy to do with our health and well-being. Sometimes, the search can feel overwhelming because it does not always exist—especially regarding the human body, health, building strength, and managing pain. We are complex, dynamic creatures who often require complex and dynamic paths to feeling confident and aging strong. No "one-size-fits-all" solution exists. The positive side, though, is this provides room for many different pathways to succeed.

For Jim and many others, breaking the cycle of negative self-talk and perception is a fundamental first step to understanding the path to a resilient self.

I CAN'T DO THAT: CATASTROPHIZING AND MAGNIFICATION

Sarah was overwhelmed with anxiety as she stepped into my office. It had been about ten years since the "incident" and she was having a back pain flare this week. Although she described her pain as "mild tightness," the thought of it progressing further was terrifying. In her mind, she was right back to that day nearly a decade ago, on her kitchen floor, when she couldn't get up for hours after bending over to pick up her backpack.

As she sat down, I noticed her unease as she fidgeted in discomfort. Her tennis shoes had been slipped on with the backs folded under her heels, barefoot, and her laces untied. We started the assessment: I asked her to stand up and bend over to reach for the floor, to which she replied, "Oh, I can't do that."

Sarah voiced her frustration with her lower back and said she was worried because, after picking up a pen she had dropped yesterday, some tightness had begun to set in. She shared the events on that day in her kitchen ten years ago. "I was running late for class, bent over to pick up my backpack, and heard a pop . . . my back was stuck and I fell to the ground in pain." She had a look of defeat and fear in her eyes as she told her story. As she continued, she shared that during her recovery, she found out she had a disk herniation—and everything she read online said that bending forward and bad posture were the cause of pain like hers.

Before her back pain incident, Sarah was a carefree, active, young spitfire majoring in political science on a full-ride tennis scholarship, who loved the outdoors and lifting heavy weights. After that day, alone in her kitchen for hours, feeling fragile and hopeless, she stopped playing tennis, avoided deadlifts or any movement bending forward in the gym, and has been stuck catastrophizing the worst possible outcomes for her lower back ever since.

Sarah is not alone. This type of scenario happens all the time—an incident occurs, often traumatizing, and, from there, we create negative stories about our body.

I DON'T HAVE TIME:
REFRAMING THOUGHTS

"I can't keep up!" was Rebecca's response when I asked about roadblocks she faced to reaching her goals of feeling strong and getting back to being active.

I could sense her frustration as she talked about her "past life." Rebecca was a college swimmer. The pool was her happy place; she loved being active and had no problem prioritizing her health. Over the last fifteen years, life got "full." New corporate promotion, married to the love of her life, four kids with four different schedules . . . she was stretched pretty thin and had no place in her color-coded wall calendar for the pool, the gym, or any "Rebecca time," for that matter. "I am sick of feeling tired and achy. I know I should do more about my fitness, but I don't have time," she said with a hint of shame in her voice, as if she had let herself down.

Now, don't get me wrong, Rebecca has a busy schedule and is juggling a lot—but what if she didn't have to be? What if she reframed her thoughts and started focusing on the opportunities where pockets of time could be found, rather than on her lack of time?

CHANGING THE STORY

Our conscious brain is truly remarkable, yet 95 to 98 percent of how we show up on a daily basis is controlled by our subconscious thoughts. In other words, our actions and decisions are often a result of a pattern we're stuck in regarding the way we perceive our reality. The fact that the subconscious brain plays a vital role in how we present ourselves in daily life can feel a little overwhelming but it also creates space for opportunities to adapt your story to support the life you want to live.

Rebecca is a perfect example of this ability to adapt. At one point, it was easy and routine for her to stay active. However, priorities shifted, elements were added with career and family, and the narrative of "I am too busy" to take care of myself has been cultivated with a ton of reinforcement. This is valid—and common! Shifting these thoughts can require a lot of awareness and energy, but the opportunity to pave new pathways is there.

Jim, Sarah, and Rebecca have very different stories, but the common thread they share is the negative conviction they hold about their physical capacity. Initially, all three felt little hope or confidence about regaining their previous levels of strength and pulling out of their perceived realities. Their subconscious thoughts, molded by past experiences and ingrained beliefs, shaped their self-perception and limited their abilities.

However, by engaging in their own versions of the Belief Review and Reframe exercise (above), they overcame their resistance to change and moved forward with newfound confidence.

CHECKING IN

To build resilience within, we need to understand the power of our perception. Our minds are powerful creators, constructing our reality through the language we use to interpret our experiences. Concerning physical well-being, of course, there is a component that relates to the structure and function of *your* anatomy, but the words we choose to describe our capacity can either propel us forward or hold us back. Self-talk, characterized by statements like "I'm too old," "It's never going to get better," or "I don't have time," can set the foundation for your reality—in these examples, not a helpful one. On the other hand, positive affirmations and a reframing of thoughts, such as, "I am resilient, and I can manage this moment" can cultivate a more adaptive mindset to recover, maintain strength, and optimize physical health.

CHAPTER 2

SUPPORT, NAVIGATING STRESS, AND CREATING SAFETY

The nervous system, especially the brain, handles our thinking, memory, decision-making, and problem-solving skills.

A well-regulated autonomic nervous system ensures these cognitive functions run smoothly, which is vital for staying sharp as we age. Efficient nervous system regulation also enhances our ability to adapt, learn new skills, and build strength, all things that support physical activities by boosting coordination, reaction times, and overall performance. When we are building strength or managing pain, our autonomic nervous system needs to be able to access a sense of safety and ease to progress forward. If we are stuck in a "fight-or-flight" mode, in unmanageable, high stress all the time, the body recognizes whatever you are doing in that moment—whether it's exercise, a task, playing sports, or simply bending over to put on your socks—as a threat. Creating a safe environment in times like these and navigating stress is a crucial foundation for staying independent. When it comes to the human body, well-being, pain management, and building strength, we tend to oversimplify things, which can add to the stress.

"Your back pain is due to your glutes not firing."
"Your glutes are stiff—that's why your back hurts."

"Your joints hurt because you eat too much dairy."
"Your joints hurt because you aren't using CBD lotion."

"You need to stretch more."
"You're stretching too much."

Have you ever heard something like this and felt immediately frustrated or triggered—because for *you* it just wasn't that simple? Can these simplified ideas be helpful for some people? Absolutely. However, the moment we can shift the narrative away from the things that might be "wrong" toward a more hopeful and autonomous place is the moment we feel more empowered to manage our stress. If we can start looking at our health and well-being as a more complex and dynamic situation, we can free ourselves from the idea that *one* singular thing is the cause of the problem—or the solution. All the tools, exercises, and pieces of advice are more efficient and effective when we can regulate our nervous system and feel as though we are in a safe environment to do so.

Tips for Regulating Your Nervous System

Breathwork

- **Box breathing:** Inhale for a count of four, hold for four, exhale for four, and hold again for four.
- **Deep breathing:** Slow, deep breaths can reduce sympathetic nervous system activity (the fight-or-flight part of your nervous system) and promote relaxation.

Fuel

Eat a **balanced diet** rich in nutrients that support nervous system health, such as omega-3 fatty acids, antioxidants, and vitamins.

Meditation

Paying attention to the present moment— without judgment—can calm the mind and reduce cortisol (stress hormone) spikes. Regular practice can enhance parasympathetic nervous system (the "rest-and-recovery" part of your nervous system) activity, leading to improved emotional regulation and reduced stress.

Movement

Regular physical **exercise** and activity can help balance the sympathetic and parasympathetic nervous systems. **Yoga, stretching, and mindful movement** combine movement with breath control, promoting relaxation and nervous system balance.

Sleep Hygiene

Set up your environment to promote adequate, restful sleep to support the body's natural regulation processes.

Social Connections

Engaging in **positive social interactions** can promote happiness and reduce stress.

Therapeutic Techniques

- **Biofeedback and neurofeedback** teach you to control physiological functions by providing real-time feedback.
- **Therapy and counseling support** can help address chronic stress and anxiety, improving overall nervous system regulation.

A REGULATED NERVOUS SYSTEM

Our nervous system is integrated with every other bodily system, and it acts as an operating system for the body. The path to a regulated nervous system is not to eliminate stress— we need healthy amounts of stress to survive. However, learning to *manage stress* and regulating the nervous system are key for maintaining overall health and well-being. Finding ways to navigate stress can also help build confidence in movement and aging strong.

Our nervous system helps maintain homeostasis—our body's internal balance. It keeps our heart rate, blood pressure, digestion, breathing, and immune system in check, adjusting to what we need at any given moment. This balance is crucial for pain management and building strength by allowing our body to access energy efficiently, recover properly, and manage the hormones involved in the healing process.

The autonomic nervous system (ANS) handles our stress responses through two main branches: the sympathetic nervous system (SNS) and the parasympathetic nervous system (PNS).

- The SNS kicks in during stressful times, giving us the fight-or-flight response.
- The PNS helps us relax and recover from that stress.

Proper regulation of these systems is essential for pain management. When your body can regulate the highs and lows efficiently, you recover better; you are able to recognize a stress response and recover from it with more grace. It's worth remembering that stress is not the problem. Stress is actually a good thing and a critical part of growth as a human being. Without stress, we are never challenged or presented with opportunities to evolve. The problem, however, occurs when our ability to navigate stress is compromised. If we get stuck where our nervous system shows up in only one way (in sympathetic fight-or-flight mode, or parasympathetic rest-and-recovery state) for too long, we will have trouble autocorrecting to homeostasis, and the body does not have the capacity for being in one state for long periods of time.

Our emotions are also linked tightly to the nervous system, which helps us process and respond to emotional stimuli that affect our mood and stress levels. Good emotional regulation means better mental health and overall well-being, which directly affects our physical health.

Pain is a sure way to spike a stress response. This is why the phrase from the 2000s fitness space, "No pain, no gain," is so aggravating. You may still hear this regarding getting a deep tissue massage, or stretching, or foam rolling. The reality is, that these "no pain, no gain" activities might yield a temporary state change that seems like relief, but what actually happens is a reinforcement to the nervous system and brain that this is a stressful environment. If you want results, for many people, doing the exact opposite is effective. For example: creating a safe environment for movement, receiving a lighter-touch massage that doesn't put you further into a pain response, or checking in with yourself and modifying exercises to continue loading the painful area in a way that actually feels good.

CHALLENGE SAFELY

Challenging our body's capacities while also reinforcing safety is key when teaching our nervous systems to relax. I will give you an example. You have super-tight hips and you decide you will do whatever it takes to "loosen" them up. Maybe you grit your teeth through a foam-rolling session, tell your massage therapist to push harder because you have a high pain tolerance, and then hold a few stretches that leave you feeling like your leg might rip off . . . sound familiar? Do these sound like activities that reinforce safety? Probably not. More does not always equal more when it comes to the human body. We need to work *with* the body and find ways to regulate pain rather than power through.

Try This: 5-4-3-2-1 Grounding Body Practice

The ability to be present and connected is an incredible tool for regulating the nervous system. When our body is overwhelmed, fatigued, or in pain, we need ways to downshift and recover. One way to do this is by connecting to our five senses. It is easy to spiral into what could happen or dwell on things in the past, especially as we age and worry about physical limitations or old injuries. By focusing on things that are true, present, and happening right now, you can pull yourself out of the past and the future and return toward homeostasis.

1. Find a quiet space.
In your chosen space, take a position that allows you to bring awareness to your body easily in an area of focus. For example, if your hips are tight, find a position such as child's pose or runner's lunge that puts the hips in a gentle stretch. Take a few deep breaths to center yourself.

2. Engage your senses.
Five things you can see: Look around and name five things you can see. Take time to observe details about each item.

Example: "I see my dog by the door, a book on the couch, the sun shining through the window, a cup of coffee, and a folded blanket in a basket."

Four things you can feel: Focus on four things you can physically feel. Notice textures, temperature, and sensations.

Example: "I feel the carpet's softness, the stretch on the outside of my hip, the cool fabric of my shorts, and the sun's warmth."

Three things you can hear: Listen carefully and identify three sounds in your environment.

Example: "I hear the air conditioner's hum, birds chirping outside, and the faint sound of traffic."

Two things you can smell: Notice two different scents around you. If you can't smell anything, think of two smells you like.

Example: "I smell the fresh coffee, and I can faintly smell the scent of a candle."

One thing you can taste: Focus on one thing you can taste. It might be a lingering taste in your mouth, or you could take a sip of a drink or eat a small snack.

Example: "I can taste the mint from my toothpaste."

3. Reflect and breathe.

Take five to seven deep breaths. How do you feel now compared to when you started the exercise? Notice any changes in your stress or anxiety levels.

CHECKING IN

There are many ways to improve mobility, strength, and resilience as we age, but spending time understanding your nervous system and how to manage the highs, lows, and transitions will help you optimize all other efforts. This is a step that many of us ignore because we are hungry for quick results, but try it: Check in with yourself, especially if you are not seeing the results you would like from parts 2 and 3 of this book. Do you feel like you have a good handle on your emotional and physical stress? Do you feel like your body has opportunities to recover? Are there safe ways you can add stimulus to your body to promote adaptation or change that you've been avoiding? Take some time with this one; I promise it is a key player and could be the change that makes all the difference for you in your "age strong" journey.

CHAPTER 3

WATER, FUEL, SLEEP

I know what you're thinking: *Where are the exercises that are going to help me reach my goals?* Whether you are looking to front-squat 300 pounds (136 kg), run a 5K, get out of a chair without flaring your back pain, or improving overall mobility so you can reach the coffee mugs on the top shelf, it is important to first assess the foundation.

I think we can underestimate the impact that adequate hydration, fuel, and sleep have on our body. As we age, the pillars of water, nutrition, and sleep become ever more crucial for maintaining strength and managing pain.

HYDRATION

Staying well hydrated is fundamental to our health. Water is vital for all our body's functions, including digestion, nutrient absorption, and circulation. As we grow older, our sense of thirst diminishes, making dehydration more likely. This can lead to issues like constipation, urinary tract infections, and impaired cognitive function. Dehydration can also exacerbate chronic pain by reducing lubrication in our joints, leading to stiffness and discomfort. Keeping hydrated is essential for joint health, ensuring our cartilage remains flexible and reducing friction that can cause pain.

TIPS FOR STAYING HYDRATED

Drink water regularly: Thirst is a late indicator of dehydration and, as we age, this indicator becomes less reliable. Drinking water regularly helps maintain optimal hydration levels. Aim to drink water consistently throughout the day, not just when you feel thirsty. A general rule is 1 ounce (30 ml) of water per pound (454 g) of body weight. If you're away from home a lot, carry a water bottle so water is readily available to drink frequently.

Set reminders: Regular reminders can help create a habit of drinking water consistently. Use phone alarms, apps, or sticky notes to remind yourself to drink water throughout the day.

Drink water before meals: Make it a habit to drink a glass of water before each meal. It can help you stay hydrated and aid digestion.

Stay hydrated during exercise: Exercise increases water loss through sweat, so replenishing fluids is crucial for performance and recovery. Drink water before, during, and after physical activity.

Limit dehydrating beverages: These types of drinks can increase urine production and fluid loss. Reducing your intake of caffeinated and alcoholic beverages, which can dehydrate you, is better for overall health.

Adjust for weather: Higher temperatures and dry air can increase fluid loss through sweat and evaporation. Increase your water intake during hot weather or when you spend time in dry environments.

Listen to your body: Being attuned to your body's signals helps you stay ahead of dehydration and maintain optimal hydration levels. Signs of dehydration include dry mouth, headache, or fatigue. Respond by drinking water.

FUEL

Nutrition and how we fuel our body also plays a key role in aging well. A balanced diet rich in essential nutrients supports overall vitality. Nutrition can be a complex topic because we have individual requirements. There is no "best" diet or most effective program or plan for aging strong. Sticking with a whole food focus, rich in a variety of micronutrients, is a great place to start.

Calcium and vitamin D are crucial for bone health, preventing osteoporosis and fractures, while omega-3 fatty acids, found in fish and flaxseed, have anti-inflammatory properties that can help manage chronic pain and are also good for brain health. Maintaining a healthy balance of protein, carbs, and fat is also key.

MACRONUTRIENTS

Macronutrients help the body function properly and include carbohydrates, protein, and fat. Fad diets, which come and go, may advise eliminating one (or more) macronutrients, but all three are important for overall health and strength. A general rule for macronutrient distribution in a balanced diet is:

- **Carbohydrates:** 50–60 percent of daily calories
- **Protein:** 25–40 percent of daily calories
- **Fats:** 20–35 percent of daily calories

These guidelines can be adjusted based on individual health goals, activity levels, dietary preferences, and specific nutritional needs. Consult with a health care provider or registered dietitian for personalized advice for optimal nutrition.

Carbohydrates

Carbohydrates provide fuel and quick energy for our body. Prioritize complex carbs that provide fiber and essential nutrients, such as whole grains, vegetables, and fruits. Limit refined sugars and highly processed options, which can spike blood sugar and lead to illness and poor health.

Protein

Protein is essential for muscle repair, immune system function, and overall body maintenance. Choose lean sources of protein when you can and vary your intake to include both animal and plant-based proteins.

Protein-Rich Foods

For many people, finding quality protein sources can be the most challenging macronutrient to keep up with. Adding these protein-rich foods to your diet can help build lean muscle as you age strong.

PROTEIN	SERVING SIZE	# OF PROTEIN GRAMS
Almonds	1 ounce (28 g), about 23 almonds	6 grams
Black Beans	1 cup (172 g) cooked	15 grams
Chicken Breast	3 ounces (85 g)	26 grams
Eggs	2 large (100 g)	12 grams
Lentils	1 cup (198 g) cooked	18 grams
Quinoa	1 cup (185 g) cooked	8 grams
Salmon	3 ounces (85 g)	22 grams
Tuna (canned in water)	3 ounces (85 g)	20 grams

Fats

Healthy fats are crucial for brain health, hormone production, long-form energy, and nutrient absorption. When eating fats, focus on unsaturated fats found in avocados, fish, nuts, and seeds, while limiting saturated fats and avoiding trans fats.

SLEEP

Proper sleep is another fundamental for maintaining health. Quality sleep allows our body to undergo critical restorative processes, including muscle repair, memory consolidation, and the regulation of hormones that control appetite and stress. Poor sleep can disrupt these processes and, as discussed in chapter 2, managing stress is a critical part of staying strong and maintaining independence.

Adequate sleep helps manage chronic pain by reducing inflammation and expanding pain tolerance. Without adequate sleep, our perception of pain heightens and our ability to cope with it diminishes. Additionally, good sleep is essential for good mental health and reducing stress and anxiety, which can also decrease our perception of physical pain.

TIPS TO OPTIMIZE SLEEP

Pay attention to your microbiome. Your gut bacteria can greatly affect how well you sleep because they help control the production of serotonin, a chemical in your brain that influences sleep cycles. Incorporate prebiotics and probiotics into your diet. Foods such as fiber-rich vegetables, kefir, sauerkraut, and yogurt can improve gut health and, subsequently, enhance sleep quality.

Light exposure matters. The timing of light exposure influences our circadian rhythm, which regulates sleep-wake cycles. Morning light exposure is particularly beneficial. Try to get at least thirty minutes of natural sunlight exposure within the first hour of waking. This practice helps regulate your internal clock and improve nighttime sleep quality.

Regulate body temperature. Core body temperature naturally decreases during sleep. Enhancing this natural drop can promote deeper, more restorative sleep. Consider taking a warm bath or shower 1 to 2 hours before bedtime. The subsequent cooling down after the bath helps lower core body temperature, signaling to your body that it's time to sleep.

Time meals and snacks for your best sleep. When you eat your last meal or snack before bedtime can significantly impact sleep quality. Eating too close to bedtime can interfere with the body's natural sleep processes. When possible, finish eating at least 2 to 3 hours before going to bed. This allows your body to complete the digestion process and prevents discomfort or acid reflux that can disrupt sleep. Additionally, avoid heavy, spicy, or high-sugar foods in the evening, as these can negatively affect sleep quality. If you need something before bed, choose a light, protein-rich snack, such as a small serving of yogurt or a handful of nuts.

Cultivate your sound environment. Consistent, soothing sounds can enhance sleep by masking disruptive noises and promoting relaxation. Use white or pink noise machines, which can improve sleep quality by creating a consistent sound environment and help mask sudden noises that might disturb sleep.

If you feel overwhelmed or concerned with the quality of your hydration, nutrition, or sleep habits, consult a professional who can help you navigate these important areas based on your current goals and health status. Prioritizing these aspects can enhance your quality of life, reduce the risk of chronic conditions, and maintain independence and vitality.

Try This: Progressive Muscle Relaxation Journal Exercise for Sleep

Progressive muscle relaxation (PMR) helps reduce physical tension and promote relaxation, leading to better sleep. This journal exercise guides you through incorporating PMR into your nightly routine and tracking its effect on your sleep quality. This way, you can identify what works best for your sleep routine and make informed adjustments to achieve better rest and support overall well-being.

1. Find a quiet, comfortable place to lie down. Close your eyes and take a few deep breaths.
2. Starting from your feet and working up to your head, tense each muscle group for 5 to 10 seconds, then relax for 20 to 30 seconds. Focus on the feeling of relaxation in each muscle group before moving to the next.
   - Feet: Curl your toes tightly, then release.
   - Legs: Tighten your calves and thighs, then release.
   - Abdomen: Suck in your stomach, then release.
   - Hands and arms: Clench your fists and tighten your arms, then release.
   - Shoulders: Shrug your shoulders up to your ears, then release.
   - Face: Scrunch your facial muscles, then release.
3. The next morning, record the time you practiced PMR the night before and the session's duration. Note any immediate effects or feelings of relaxation you experienced.
4. Track your bedtime, wake-up time, total sleep duration, and sleep quality. Rate your sleep quality on a scale of 1 to 5 (1 = very poor, 5 = excellent).
5. Note any sleep disturbances or wakeups during the night. Reflect on how PMR affects your sleep and any changes you feel.
6. Each week, review your daily PMR logs to identify patterns or improvements in sleep quality. Look for correlations between PMR practice and changes in sleep disturbances or overall relaxation.
7. Based on your reflections, set specific goals for the upcoming week, such as increasing the duration of PMR sessions or ensuring you practice PMR at the same time each night.

CHECKING IN

Hydration, how we nourish our bodies, and the quality of sleep we get play a direct role in our ability to build muscle, heal from injuries, and continue to age stronger. Because it is sometimes more difficult to see the direct correlation between these three foundational pillars of health and our ability to move well and feel confident as we progress through life, we often disassociate the impact they can have. If you are like most people, I know you are eager to progress to parts 2 and 3 to learn more about the exercises that will support your mobility and strength goals, but if you feel like one of the areas covered in part 1 is lacking attention, I promise that you won't regret focusing on that first or at least in conjunction with what comes next. Spend time with this chapter (even 2 to 3 months) and choose one area to work on at a time, building strong habits there. Keep a journal to track variables you adjust and how the work has made a difference in your overall well-being.

CHAPTER 4

HUMAN CONNECTION AND RELATIONSHIPS

"I really am trying to make some lifestyle changes, but every time I work out, my back flares. I wish I had friends or people I knew who could keep me accountable and introduce me to different ways to stay active. I feel stuck! I am so ready to stop hurting all the time."

Larissa had just moved—a new city, new job, new beginning. She had just gone through a break-up, leaving her entire social circle behind, and was feeling lost, missing the safety net of her old life, but she knew it was time for a fresh start.

The only opportunity for connection with the people from her past was through happy hours, pub hopping, or weekend getaways. Part of her new beginning was also stepping into a healthier lifestyle, but she felt stuck and alone.

Be Aware! Factors That Can Affect Social Wellness

- Change in ability
- Change in job
- Death of a partner
- Depression
- Fear
- Illness
- Relocation
- Retirement

Larissa soon realized that she needed to put herself in situations where she could build community with people aligned with the direction she wanted to go. After months of putting herself out there, attending local events, meeting new faces, and engaging in different activities, she started to form a new network.

Connecting Socially Through Movement

- Attend charity walks or fitness events
- Connect with local groups building community around movement
- Find free yoga in the park or run clubs
- Join a community-focused local gym
- Learn a new sport like golf, pickleball, tennis, or water aerobics

Her determination to create a new life was inspiring and had me reflecting on how much value there is in establishing a sense of connection. If you think about it, so much of how we spend our time and resources is dependent on this sense of connection. It's why we are attracted to the clothes we purchase, the coffee shops we support, the gyms we go to, the content we consume . . . it is no different for aging stronger.

Building your foundation for health and well-being, finding your people, fostering those human connections, and cultivating relationships is one of the most important—and overlooked—parts of wellness. Relationships are a "basic need" for aging with resilience.

Longevity is another benefit of strong relationships. Studies have shown that people with strong social connections have lower mortality rates, as emotional support helps individuals cope with health challenges more effectively. Positive relationships enhance the quality of life by providing companionship, reducing loneliness, and promoting a sense of purpose and fulfillment.

A 2010 meta-analysis of 148 studies with more than 300,000 participants reviewed the connection between social relationships and mortality risk. The conclusion stated that individuals with strong social relationships had a 50 percent increased likelihood of survival compared to those with weaker social connections. This effect was comparable to other established risk factors for mortality, such as smoking and alcohol consumption. The comprehensive analysis highlights that social relationships should be regarded as a critical factor in health outcomes and vitality, similar to other well-recognized risk factors.

Another systematic review, "Social Participation and Health: A Cross-Sectional Study Among Older Adults in Norway," published in *BMC Public Health*, investigates the relationship between social participation and health among older adults. This study reviews research that explores how various forms of social participation affect physical and mental health outcomes. The study finds that higher levels of social participation are significantly associated with better physical and mental health. Older adults who frequently engage in social activities report better overall health, lower levels of depression, and higher life satisfaction. Different types of social activities, such as volunteer work, attending social gatherings, and participating in organized groups, all contribute positively to health by providing a sense of purpose, increasing physical activity levels, and fostering social relationships. The findings suggest that promoting social participation among older adults can effectively enhance their health and well-being.

Tips for Staying Connected and Building Community

Join local clubs or groups that match your interests, such as book clubs, gardening clubs, or hobby groups. Regularly attending meetings and events builds a sense of community and fosters new friendships.

Volunteer for local charities, schools, or community organizations. Volunteering provides a sense of purpose and connects you with others who share similar values.

Attend community events, such as festivals, fairs, and cultural events, where you can engage with your community.

Join group exercise classes, such as yoga, tai chi, or strength training, which not only improve physical health but also provide social interaction and support.

Take up a new skill or hobby or re-learn an old one that involves group participation, such as dancing, painting, or cooking. Shared interests can lead to meaningful connections and friendships.

Maintain regular contact with loved ones— schedule regular phone calls, video chats, or visits with family and friends. Consistent communication strengthens bonds and provides emotional support.

Attend educational workshops, seminars, or lectures on topics that interest you. Learning in a group setting can lead to new friendships and professional connections.

Join online communities, such as online forums, discussion groups, or social media communities, that expose you to more things that interest you. Online communities provide opportunities to connect with like-minded individuals, share knowledge, and find support, especially if in-person interactions are limited.

Travel with friends or family. Shared experiences and adventures strengthen bonds and create lasting memories.

Engage in intergenerational activities, such as mentoring programs, family reunions, or community or school projects. Interacting with people of various ages broadens your perspective and enhances your sense of community.

A solid network is important to maintaining independence as we age; however, building strong social circles provides both physical and emotional support at any age. Being with people and creating deep connections with others is powerful. Sure, it's nice to have friends and family around to hold you accountable, to support you with your goals, and even join you in your activities, but the real benefits come with regular social interactions that prevent isolation and loneliness. Being connected increases cognitive function, combats feelings of depression, and can instill a sense of purpose and belonging. Engaging in social activities, volunteer work, and hobbies keeps individuals physically and mentally active and connected to their communities, contributing to a positive outlook on life.

The relationship between human connections and overall health is profound and multifaceted. Strong social connections also play a vital role in encouraging healthy behaviors.

This is why certain circles in health and fitness have been so successful over the years. If you ask anyone who participates in CrossFit what they love most about their gym, most will mention the people, the friends they have made, and the connections they have built. Building community around movement brings people together. People show up for the desired outcomes and stay for the people.

Try This: Who Are You? What Lights You Up?

Life can get so full—with work, family, and other people's expectations—we lose sight of who we are and what we love. Pull out a journal and try this exercise.

Part 1: Self-Reflection

Answer the following questions:
- What are your best qualities?
- What lights you up when you're at your best?
- How can you add more of that into your life?
- What are your personal core values?

Part 2: Find Your Tribe

On one page in your journal, make four lists with these four headings:
1. **Personal connections** (people you know personally and value most)
2. **Role models** (those you look up to, but might not know personally)
3. **Communities** (alumni, church, digital, gym, physical, work, etc.)
4. **Content** (ideas/thoughts/insights delivered to you and created by others)

Part 3: Connecting the Dots

On a second page, put your name in a bubble in the center, and web out three to eight bubbles that include your main core values from part 1. Go back to your list from part 2 and connect lines from your core value bubbles to the corresponding people, communities, and content.

Part 4: Reflection

For some people, it will be easy to connect your core values to the people and content from part 2; for others, it will be difficult. This self-reflection is meant to be an audit of who and what you spend your time and energy on. If you have core values that are empty, what can you do to fill in those blanks? If you have people, communities, or content that don't match up to any of your core values, ask yourself: How they are serving you?

CHECKING IN

Positive relationships are fostered when they match your core values. These connections provide emotional support, reduce stress, and lead to improved health and happiness. By investing in strong social connections, you can enjoy a healthier, more fulfilling life and age stronger, maintaining both physical and mental well-being.

PART 2

Whole Body Movements

CHAPTER 5

SIT TO STAND

"I'm scared to sit back on my couch—it took me over half an hour to get up! I'm too young to need help sitting up." My patient, frustrated with an old back injury, told me this, then burst into tears when she relayed how it was affecting her daily life.

Maintaining the ability to transition from sitting to standing is a cornerstone of independence and daily functionality as we age. This movement is integral to many everyday activities—from getting out of a car and rising from a chair to standing up from the toilet and participating in social gatherings. Without the strength, mobility, and control to perform this fundamental action, our quality of life can significantly diminish, along with our physical and emotional well-being.

You may wonder, *"How would I get to the point where I can't perform simple tasks like getting off the couch?"* Our convenient lifestyles encourage complacency in how we carry ourselves throughout the day. To maintain strength and mobility, however, we need to continue to find opportunities to challenge our bodies.

Beyond the physical benefits, the ability to transition smoothly from sitting to standing enables people to maintain autonomy—to perform daily tasks independently without relying on others for help. This autonomy is vital to preserving self-esteem and fostering confidence, which are crucial for overall mental health.

Note The movements in this chapter build strength, mobility, and control in the body. Find a movement variation that feels good in your body and doesn't produce pain. If you need to hold on to a table or chair for support on the way down into the squat, for example, do it! The goal is to build confidence and autonomy with movement.

Try This: 30-Second Chair Stand Test

Perform a light warm-up, such as marching in place, to prepare your muscles.

1. Place a stable chair without wheels, preferably with a straight back and no armrests, against a wall or a stable surface to prevent it from moving. Sit in the middle of the chair, back straight, feet flat on the floor slightly wider than hip-width apart, arms crossed over your chest, knees bent at a 90-degree angle.
2. Stand up fully to an upright position, using your legs—not your hands for support. Lower yourself back into the chair in a controlled manner, sitting down gently without plopping.
3. Continue to sit down and stand up (1 rep) as many times as you can within 30 seconds.
4. Check in:
   - How many reps did you complete within 30 seconds?
   - Ensure you are using your leg muscles to stand, sit, and maintain control throughout the movement.
   - Pay attention to your balance and whether you feel unsteady or need to use your hands for support.
   - Note any discomfort, joint stiffness, or pain in your ankles, knees, hips, or lower back.

STRENGTH

As we age, muscle mass naturally decreases, leading to muscle atrophy. Consistent strength training counters this process by promoting muscle growth and maintenance.

Incorporating targeted strength exercises into your routine is a proactive approach to aging strong. It enhances overall strength, balance, and stability significantly, all vital for preventing falls and injuries during the transition from sitting to standing, and helps preserve your independence and overall quality of life and ability to move confidently and safely. Committing to these strength exercises is an investment in your long-term physical and emotional health and empowering aging with resilience.

 Safety First If you have an injury or medical condition—especially with your hips, knees, or lower back—consult your health care provider before undertaking these exercises.

EXERCISES FOR STRENGTH

Exercises such as Chair/Box Squats (to the right) and Wall Sits (page 36) enhance the strength of our hips and legs, making it easier to stand from a sitting position safely and efficiently. These exercises focus on improving endurance in these core and leg muscles, ensuring they can move freely without pain.

Where Should I Feel It?

These movements focus on the muscles that support the hips and knees. You will feel the quadriceps and the hip flexors working hard to support your body.

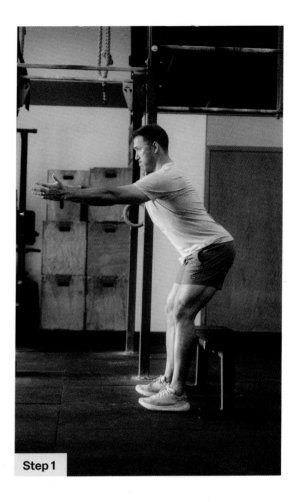

Step 1

EXERCISE 1

Chair/Box Squats

This exercise targets the same muscles used during sit-to-stand activities, like getting up from the table. Use a dining room chair, firm bench, or box from the gym to perform this exercise. And don't worry, this exercise is easy to adjust to your current capacity while you build strength (see Modifications, page 34).

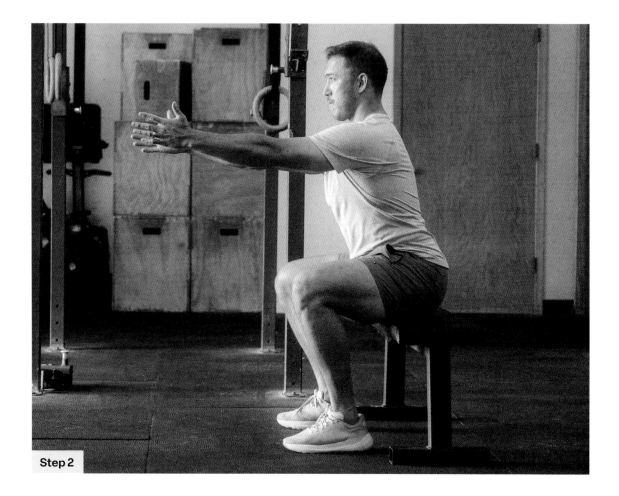

Step 2

Step 1

Stand about 6 inches (15 cm) in front of a sturdy/stable chair facing out, feet slightly wider than hip-width apart. Hinge your hips back while simultaneously counterweighting your arms forward.

Step 2

Bend your knees and lower your body down onto the chair. Keep the tension on the back side of your body along the hamstrings and glute muscles to maintain a solid foundation for the pelvis and spine. The next exercise gets you up from the chair.

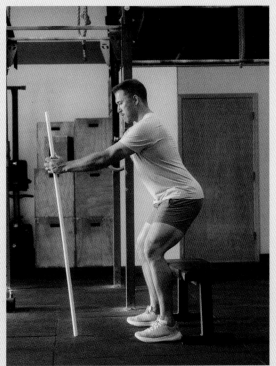

MODIFICATIONS

If you experience back pain while sitting or don't trust your balance while hinging back and down, place your chair near a table or countertop to hold onto. As you practice this movement, you'll need less support. You can also use a sturdy broomstick or pole for support.

Try different chair heights to change the distance to the target and range of motion required (more distance equals more challenge; less distance means a lesser challenge and a feeling of safety). Or place pillows, cushions, or folded blankets on the seat. As you build strength, remove the bolsters to increase capacity.

To progress this movement, add load: Hold a kettlebell at your chest, or one dumbbell in each hand down to your sides in a suitcase position (see page 80).

EXERCISE 2

Standing from Sitting

Once down onto the chair, for some, getting back up is the challenge. We stand up from a sitting position multiple times a day, so building strength for this movement is critical for maintaining independence as we age.

Step 1

From a sitting position, keep your spine tall. Widen your feet to slightly wider than hip width. Hinge your torso forward to find tension on the back side of your body.

Step 2

Reach your arms forward to counterweight your hips and lower body. Drive your weight through your heels and raise your body off the chair to a standing position.

Step 3

Repeat Chair/Box Squats and Standing from Sitting 8 to 10 times.

MODIFICATIONS

While building strength, use a table in front of you to support your body weight as you transition from sitting to standing, and standing to sitting. As your strength grows, use the prop less.

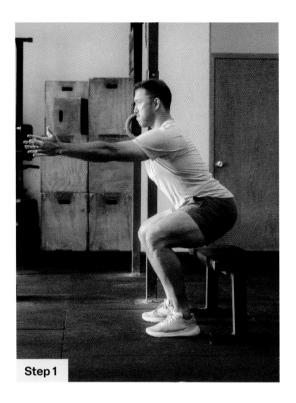

Step 1

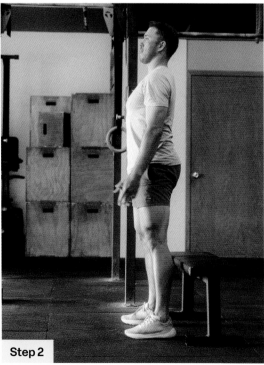

Step 2

EXERCISE 3

Wall Sit

This exercise builds isometric endurance in the muscles that support the hips and the spine. Taking a potentially challenging dynamic activity, like sitting to standing, dissecting it, and turning it into an isometric exercise can create confidence and trust in performing the activity.

Step 1

Stand with your back against the wall, feet about hip-width apart. While bending your knees, slowly lower yourself into a sitting position, back still against the wall, knees bent at about a 90-degree angle. Don't obsess about the exact positioning of your knees or feet—concentrate on finding a "seated" position that challenges the leg and hip muscles. Hold for 20 seconds, or more if you can.

Step 2

To get out of this position, push down into your feet to slide up the wall to a standing position, or put your hands on your knees and push yourself up to standing.

Step 3

Repeat 3 to 5 times, aiming to hold for the same duration each time.

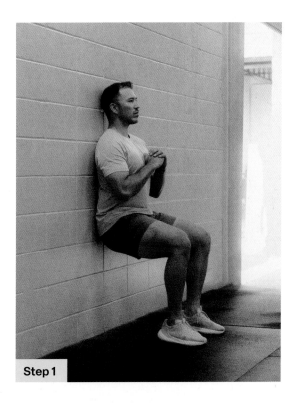

Step 1

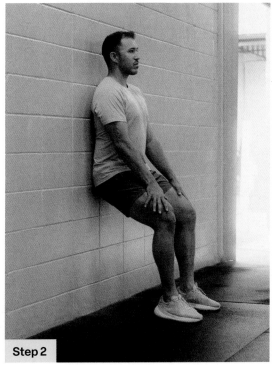

Step 2

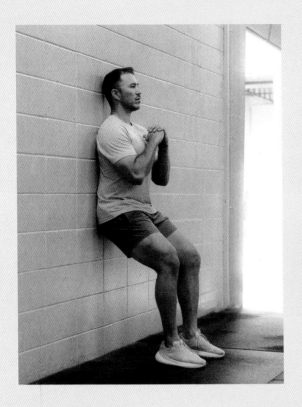

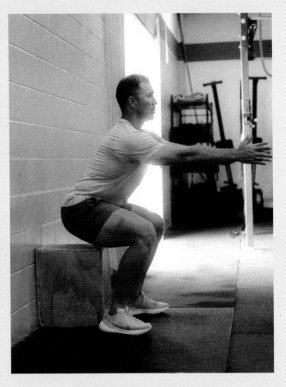

MODIFICATION 1

If this feels difficult, slide up the wall so you are not so deep in the squat position, which takes some bend out of your knees to put less demand on your legs.

MODIFICATION 2

If you have the strength but don't trust yourself in the wall sit or squat position, place a small bench or stool against the wall for support and hover above it in a wall-sit position. As you become stronger, decrease the stool's height or increase the time held in the exercise.

EXERCISE 4

Wall Sit with Hinge

To bridge the gap between the Wall Sit (page 36) and Standing from Sitting (page 35), work in a hinge from the wall-sit position.

Step 1

Following step 1 of the Wall Sit (page 36), set up into a wall-sit position.

Step 2

Pull your upper back off the wall and drive tension through the hips into the wall as if you are bowing forward, ending with your torso at about a 45-degree angle from the floor.

Step 3

Pull your chest away from the floor, bringing your torso to the upright position to complete a full repetition. Go slowly—take about 2 seconds to get into the bow and 2 seconds to come back up.

Step 4

Repeat 6 to 8 times.

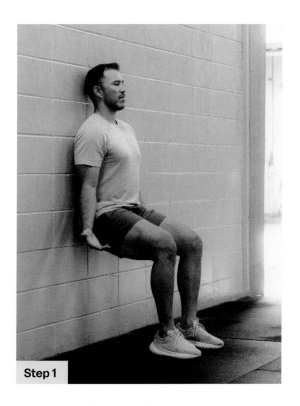
Step 1

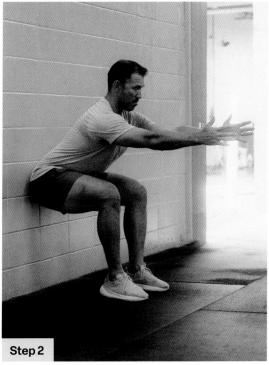
Step 2

MOBILITY

Of course, there are reasons people become stiffer as they age, such as certain chronic conditions, genetic components, and history of accidents or trauma, but mostly it results from lack of movement. Most of us adopt repetitive patterns, postures, and positions: sitting for hours, and spending the majority of our day on our phones or laptops. Most jobs keep us fairly sedentary, which means we have to be intentional about moving our bodies in a variety of ways to maintain joint health, mobility, and range of motion. Alongside strength, prioritizing mobility in the hips, knees, and ankles will make getting up from a seated position more efficient.

EXERCISES FOR MOBILITY

These exercises offer ways to expose the hips, knees, and ankles to more range of motion in a safe way. These exercises are focused more on the joints rather than stretching the surrounding muscles like the glutes, quads, hamstrings, and calf muscles. Sure, you may feel a stretching sensation in these areas during these exercises, but the goal is safe and confident mobility in the joints.

Where Should I Feel It?

You may feel stiffness or resistance in the spine, hips, knees, and ankle joints. Remember, working through some resistance in a way that feels safe and productive can be okay, but working through pain is not. If any movement causes pain, try the modifications or consult with your care provider.

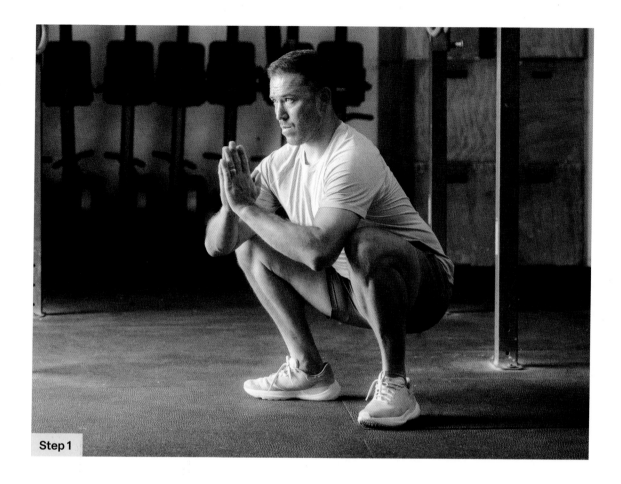

Step 1

EXERCISE 5

Deep Squat
(Hip/Knee/Ankle)

The deep squat exposes the hips, knees, and ankles to end range of motion (in this case, flexion) in a safe manner, which is, ultimately, the best way to improve their mobility. Spending time in a deep squat will cultivate more range in your joints while transitioning from sitting to standing.

Step 1

Stand with your feet about two times wider than hip-width apart. Turn your toes out slightly to an angle that feels like it will allow you to drop safely into a squat. Drop into a deep squat, sitting your hips as low as you can. It is okay if your heels come off the ground for this exercise—the goal is to get into the most ankle, knee, and hip flexion as the body safely can.

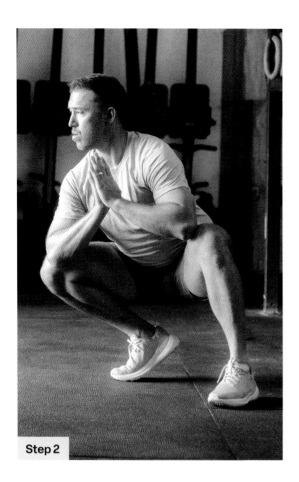

Step 2

MODIFICATIONS

If you need support to bring your center of gravity farther back to get deeper into the squat, or to come up and out of the deep squat, hold on to a counter, table, or chair. The main goal with this movement is to get the hips, knees, and ankles exposed to deep flexion and sometimes this can be very challenging without offloading some body weight. Using your upper body strength to adjust how much bodyweight you are loading your joints with can be a great way to build capacity in the joints of the lower body involved in squatting.

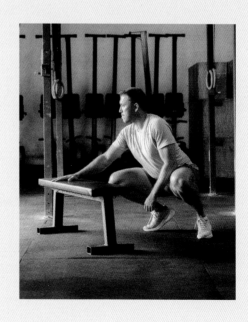

Step 2

Shift your weight to one side for 3 to 5 seconds to increase ankle and knee flexion, then shift to the other side for 3 to 5 seconds. Repeat 2 to 3 times on each side.

Step 3

Come back to center, press through the ground, and stand up tall.

EXERCISE 6

Elevated Front Foot Split Squat

This squat, like the Deep Squat (page 40), also exposes the hip, knee, and ankle joints to their end range of motion. Doing this in a split stance, though, isolates one leg at a time and creates a more trusted environment for the body to drop into. You can elevate the front foot for this in many ways: at the gym on a box or a barbell plate, or at home on a stool or even the bottom step of a staircase. This makes deep flexion feel more approachable because there's less stress on the knee joint.

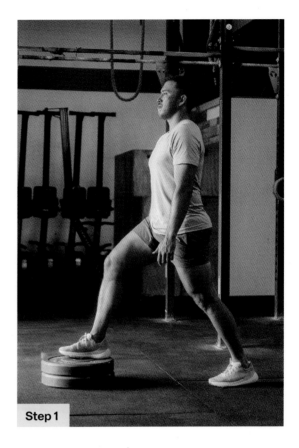

Step 1

Step 1

Place a prop 8 to 10 inches (20 to 25 cm) high (yoga block, sturdy stepstool, or box) on the floor in front of you. Place your front (right) foot on the prop and take a big step back, slightly farther than a walking stride, with the other (left) foot.

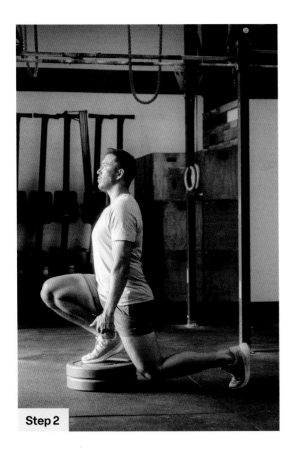

Step 2

MODIFICATIONS

If you're struggling, raise the prop's height until it feels tolerable and safe to find deep flexion in the knee and ankle. As this exercise gets less challenging, adjust the variables: Add weight by holding dumbbells in both hands down to your sides, reduce the height of the prop under the front foot, or change the exercise tempo.

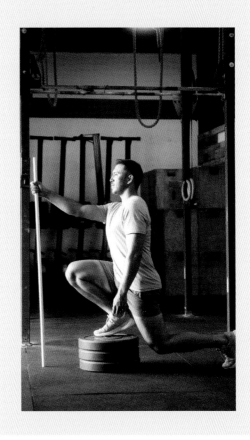

Step 2
Drive your front (right) knee forward over your toes, bringing your knee and ankle into deep flexion. Hold for 3 to 5 seconds. Don't worry if the heel comes off the raised surface—the goal is finding maximum pain-free flexion of the knee and ankle.

Step 3
Return to the starting position and repeat on the same side 4 to 6 times.

Step 4
Repeat on the other side.

BALANCE AND CONTROL

Alongside strength and mobility training to support getting in and out of a seated position, you also can work on balance and joint control. Having the necessary balance and joint control not only keeps you feeling independent navigating daily activities, but also helps prevent falls.

EXERCISES FOR BALANCE AND CONTROL

These exercises build balance and joint control via adjusting the movement's tempo by either increasing the time under tension or slowing things to a static hold. The more we can challenge this type of activity in diverse ways, the more trust we build in completing the movement.

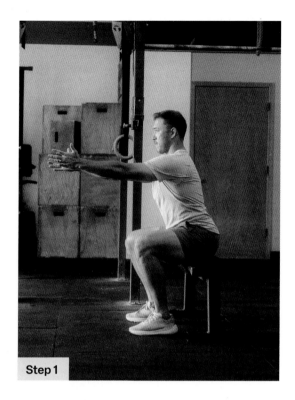

Step 1

Where Should I Feel It?

You will feel this in the hip flexors, hamstrings, glutes, and all the muscles that support the hip joint. Building endurance in these activities can lead to muscle fatigue but should not feel pinch-y or painful. If it does, try a modification.

EXERCISE 7

Squat Hover

Similar to strength building with the Wall Sit (page 36), isometric exercises build capacity in muscles. The Squat Hover, however, removes the wall as support and demands more muscle control and endurance. This builds stability and balance in a squat position.

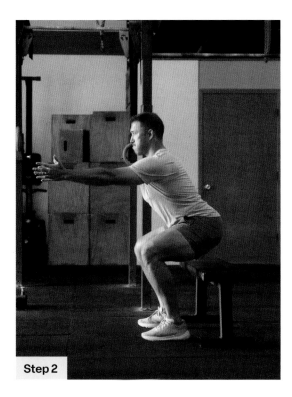

Step 2

MODIFICATIONS

Decrease the demand by raising the prop's height. To advance this exercise, increase time under tension on the way down into the squat, building the eccentric capacity of the leg muscles that help with control and balance during the transition from standing to sitting.

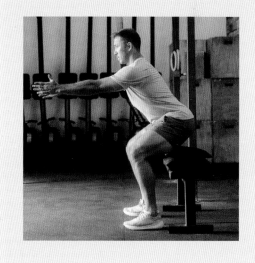

Step 1

Find a stool or sturdy box about the same height that you can squat comfortably. For example, if chair height is as deep as you feel confident squatting, use a chair as your prop. If squatting deeper is your challenge, use a shorter prop. Stand in front of the prop with your feet slightly wider than hip-width apart and squat down to the prop as you would when doing a Chair/Box Squat (page 32).

Step 2

Lift your sit bones off the prop and hover to build static endurance. Hold. Any amount of time will start building control—aim for 15 to 20 seconds and build from there. Repeat 3 to 5 times, aiming to hold for the same duration each time.

CHECKING IN

Perform these exercises for a month or so to build strength, mobility, balance, and control. How are feeling? Are the exercises getting easier? Do you notice a change in daily activities, like getting up from the couch or sitting at your desk? Perform the 30-Second Chair Stand Test (page 31) regularly, such as once a month, to monitor your progress—and give yourself credit for making your health a priority. Keep up the good work!

CHAPTER 6

GET UP OFF THE FLOOR

"I just want to get down on the floor and play with my kids/grandkids."
"I don't get down to clean under the table because I'm not sure I can get back up."
"I love gardening, but I am nervous about falling when I try to get up."

These are common conversations I have with patients in my office.

As a child, you effortlessly moved from position to position—whether sitting on the ground, jumping to your feet, or crawling under tables. However, somewhere along the line, we start spending less time on the floor. Why is that?

I think, in part, it's that modern life provides many (perhaps too many) convenient tools—whether they're comfy couches we sink into, high tables with barstools we slide on to, or desks we adjust to our desired height—with the result being fewer reasons to be on the ground, and naturally less time spent sitting on and getting up off the ground. Over time, as our bodies lose exposure to certain movements, we also lose the ability to perform them.

Getting up off the floor is more than just a functional skill to maintain; it's also a measure of strength, mobility, and balance—three important indicators of aging strong.

Note It is perfectly acceptable to find different ways to support your body weight or modify movements. It is better to do a movement with modification than to compromise your safety.

Try This: Sit-to-Stand Test

This test determines your ability to get up off the floor unassisted, evaluating lower body strength, mobility, and control—all crucial for the task.

1. Sit on the floor, legs crossed, or in a comfortable seated position, with arms relaxed, either at your sides or crossed over your chest.
2. Without using your hands, arms, or any prop for support, stand up from the seated position, noting any difficulty, imbalance, or need for assistance that you feel.

Scoring
- If you can rise to a standing position smoothly and without assistance, you pass.
- If you use your hands, knees, or any prop for support, note the points of difficulty.

Assess
- If you did not need assistance, was there a moment when you thought you might?
- Did the movement feel smooth?
- Was this test painful? If so, where?

STRENGTH

Transitioning to and from the floor requires significant trunk strength. It challenges the muscles that support the hip joints, as well as the deep core muscles. We learn that sit-ups build a strong core, and bridges and clamshells build strong glutes. I am a firm believer that there are no good or bad movements, only unprepared ones. If your goal is being able to get on to and off the floor, sit-ups and clamshells are not the most effective preparation. Instead, finding a set of movements or exercises to better prepare you for the desired outcome, in this case getting up off the floor, is.

The neuromuscular system is a massive intricate network, more complex than we give it credit for. To provide perspective, the body works as a whole system. You use your core muscles to keep you upright, when you transition from position to position, when you walk, when you roll over in bed, and when you get off the toilet. It's the same with your glute muscles—they are "on" when you walk, when you climb stairs, when you go from a kneeling position to standing. They are always working. We just need to condition them in ways that leave us feeling prepared for the activities we desire to do.

Safety First If you have an injury or medical condition—especially with the knees, hips, or lower back—consult your health care provider before undertaking these exercises.

EXERCISES FOR STRENGTH

The following exercises help you build the strength required for getting on to, then up and off the floor.

Where Should I Feel It?

For the strength-focused exercises when you are stepping backward and standing up, you'll feel the movement in the back of the legs, specifically the hamstrings and glute muscles. You will feel the kneeling to standing exercises in the hips and throughout your core.

EXERCISE 1

Reverse Lunge with Reach

This exercise from Dr. Eric Goodman's work with Foundation Training brings in principles of counterweighting bodyweight while transitioning from standing to the floor. It helps you feel strong and confident getting to the ground. There are many ways to do this, but stepping back into a reverse lunge, then into a half-kneeling position, is typically the most approachable way.

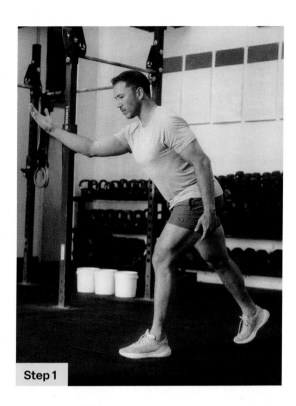

Step 1

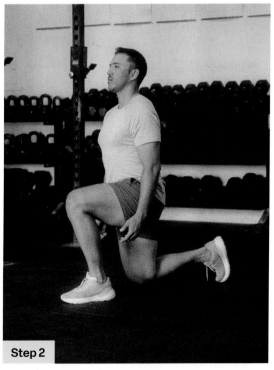

Step 2

Step 1

Stand strong on both feet, feet slightly wider than shoulder-width apart. Step backward with one foot, hinge your hips back, and, as you step, simultaneously reach the arm from the same side forward to counterweight your body.

Step 2

Bring your outstretched arm down to your side and bring your torso over your hips, finding a tall half-kneeling position, with your knee resting on the floor. The next exercise gets you up and out of this position!

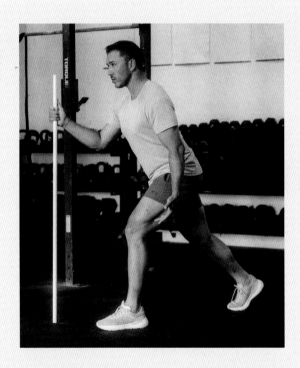

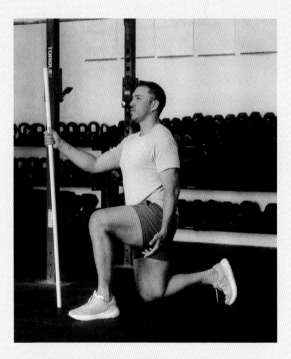

MODIFICATION 1

If your balance is in doubt as your step back and down, grab a sturdy dowel or stick for support, like a walking stick, in the hand on the same side as your leg stepping back, or place yourself next to a sturdy structure to hold onto to assist you to the floor.

MODIFICATION 2

If it's too uncomfortable to put your knee on the floor, place a towel, pillow, or pad underneath it.

EXERCISE 2

Step with Reach to Standing

The next objective is being able to reverse out of the Reverse Lunge with Reach (page 48) back to standing. This requires strength and control in the front leg to support your body weight from the floor to a standing position.

Step 1

From the half-kneeling position, hinge your hips back slightly and simultaneously reach your arm (on the same side as the knee on the floor) forward.

Step 2

Shift your weight forward, reaching with your arm, putting your center of gravity over your front (standing) foot. Drive pressure into the front foot and lift yourself up as you step your bent leg forward to meet your front leg in a standing position.

Step 3

When proficient in exercises 1 (Reverse Lunge with Reach, page 48) and 2 (Step with Reach to Standing, this page), repeat 6 to 8 times on one side, then switch to the other.

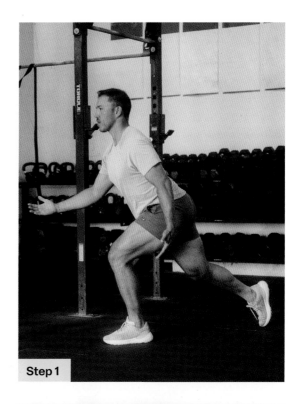

Step 1

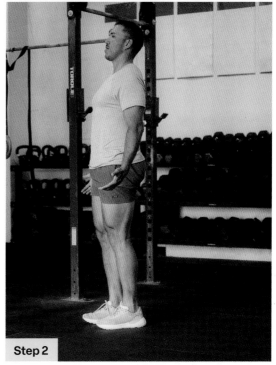

Step 2

MODIFICATIONS

If balance is an issue or you do not have the strength to lift yourself up from this position, grab a sturdy dowel or stick for support, or hold on to a countertop to assist you up off the floor.

Getting Off the Floor without Assistance

Mastering exercises 1 (Reverse Lunge with Reach, page 48) and 2 (Step with Reach to Standing, page 50) is probably all that most people need to build strength for simple tasks like cleaning, retrieving items on the ground, or playing on the floor. I've noticed, however, the challenge people experience navigating positions while on the floor, or getting up from the ground independently from a seated position.

Over the decades, longevity experts have researched the correlation between one's ability to get up and down from the floor without using upper body strength for support and mortality rates. Some study results support the idea that being able to get off the floor unassisted translates to living a longer life. In my opinion, the research I have seen on this has some holes, and there are *many* factors at play here. However, I do think this is a valuable skill and a good measure of functional strength. Conditioning your body to be more independent in any capacity is a win in my eyes.

These next two movements bridge the gap between the half-kneeling position and getting to a seated position on the floor (and back up) without using your hands.

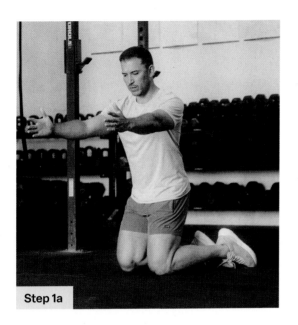

Step 1a

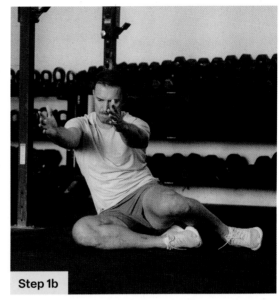

Step 1b

EXERCISE 3

Kneeling to Seated Transition

The transition from kneeling to sitting on the ground can be challenging and, again, requires significant core and hip strength. Give yourself grace and find a modification that challenges you but that you can still perform with control and without pain.

Step 1

From a tall kneeling (both knees) position, bring your lower legs and feet out to one side at about a 45-degree angle from your thighs while pulling your hips down toward the ground next to your heels. While hinging your hips back, counterweight your arms forward. This will bring you to your seat, knees bent in front of you and legs out to one side.

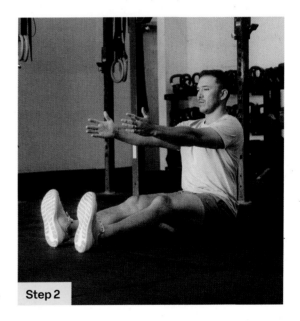

Step 2

Step 2

Unbend your knees and extend both legs straight out in front of you, sitting upright.

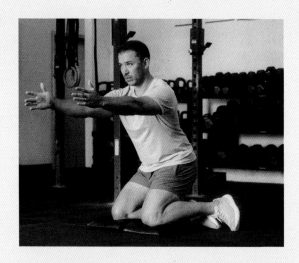

MODIFICATION 1

If you have knee pain from the pressure on the ground, place a pillow, cushion, or towel underneath your knees for support.

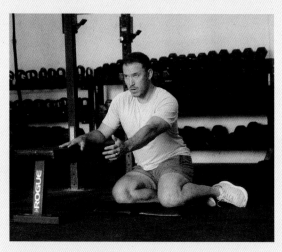

MODIFICATION 2

If you have knee pain in the bent knee while lowering yourself, or lack the hip or core strength to sit your heels down to the ground, use a sturdy dowel or bench to hold onto to gain more control with the movement. Experiment with the amount of support and gradually use less as you condition your body for this transition.

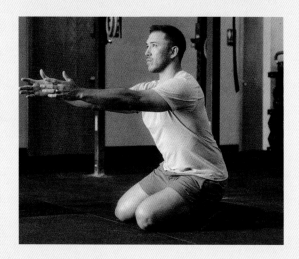

MODIFICATION 3

You can also shorten the distance to the "target" (the floor) by stacking up a few cushions or putting a pillow on a short bench where your hips land; make sure the target you choose is firm enough to support your body.

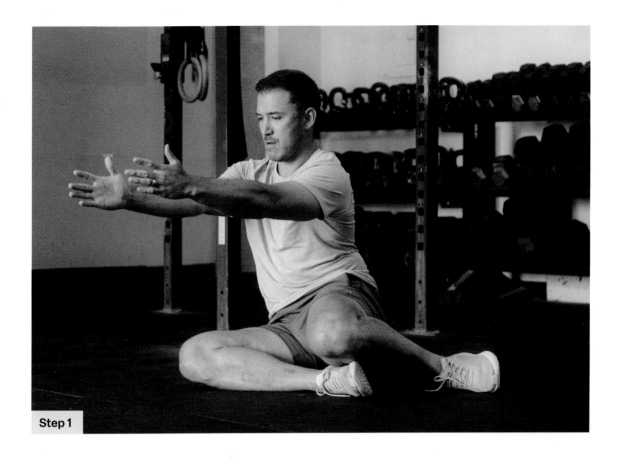

Step 1

EXERCISE 4

Sitting to Tall Kneeling Transition

When going from a seated position to the tall kneeling position, the most challenging part is usually the initial drive to get up off the ground—having enough power to lift your body weight off the floor.

Step 1

From the position in which you finished exercise 3, Kneeling to Seated Transition (page 52) (both legs straight out in front, sitting upright), bend both knees to one side and position your body as upright as possible over your hips.

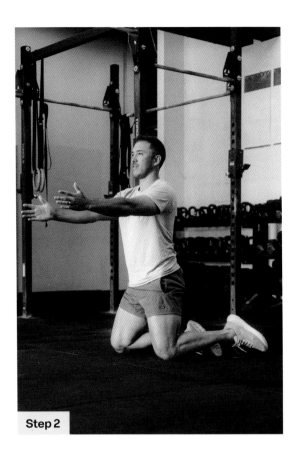

Step 2

MODIFICATIONS

If your hips feel better turned out rather than shifted to one side, start in a cross-legged position with your ankles overlapped. Rock your weight forward over your ankles into a tall kneeling position, uncross your ankles, and you will be in the tall kneeling position.

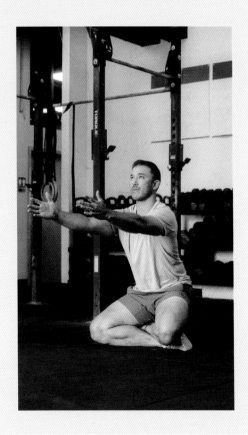

Step 2

Drive pressure into both feet as you hinge your body weight forward, controlling it up into the tall kneeling (both knees) position.

Step 3

When proficient in exercises 3 (Kneeling to Seated Transition, page 52) and 4 (Sitting to Tall Kneeling Transition, page 54), repeat 12 to 16 times, alternating which way you put your knees each time.

MOBILITY

We have established how to build strength in the hips and core to get up off the floor. The next consideration is having the mobility to support this—not flexibility or being limber—but joint *control*, which is complemented by the muscle strength-building exercises we just did. I have many patients chasing flexibility. I explain that while more range of motion can be a good thing, it also requires more responsibility. Being mobile doesn't mean much if we aren't able to control that range of motion.

EXERCISES FOR MOBILITY

These exercises build control in the hips and endurance in the spine so you feel well-equipped to get yourself down on to the floor and back up.

Where Should I Feel It?

You will feel the 90/90 Transitions with Grooving (this page) in the outside of the front leg, hip, and throughout your core. While doing the Sitting Upright on the Floor exercise (page 58), you'll feel your hip flexors and core challenged. For the Hip Hinge (page 60), you'll feel the back of the legs and spine, specifically the hamstring, glutes, and muscles in the lower back.

90/90 Transitions with Grooving

During this movement series, we will work on being on the floor and building controlled rotation in the hip joints, a range of motion typically avoided in daily movements. Typically, our daily activities involve a lot of sitting to standing to hinging to walking to running to bending—all done in one plane (frontal) of movement. We don't spend much time moving our hips side to side or in rotation, but these ranges are also important to the hip joint and helpful in getting up off the ground.

Step 1
Sit on the floor and place your legs in a 90/90, or Z, position.

Step 2
Bow your torso over the top of the front leg. When you reach the end of your range of motion in the bow, bring your torso back to an upright position. Repeat 10 to 12 times on this side.

Step 3
Repeat on the other side.

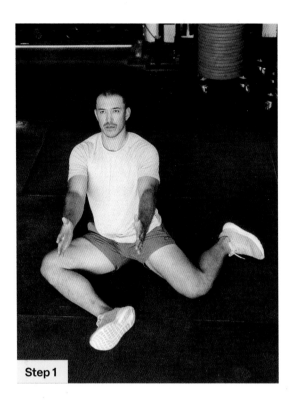

Step 1

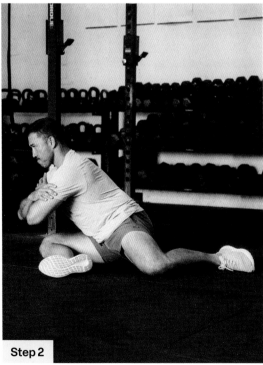

Step 2

MODIFICATIONS

If this position is not possible without pain, try sitting on a short stool or a pillow. Having a prop will change the angle that the hip sits at, potentially putting less direct stress on the joint and allowing for more opportunities to mobilize this area with confidence.

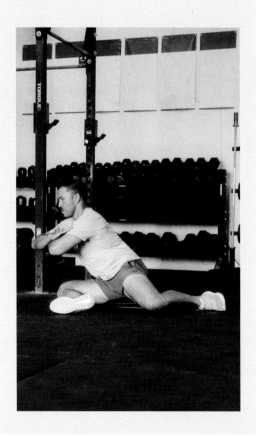

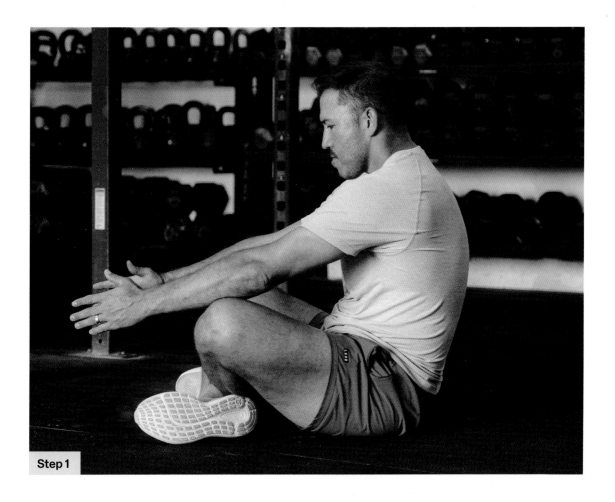

Step 1

EXERCISE 6

Sitting Upright on the Floor

At first glance, this might not seem like a mobility exercise, but in this position, we are trying to mobilize the upper back and build endurance in an upright tall position.

Step 1

Sit on the floor in a cross-legged position, as tall and upright as you can. Focus on rounding your upper back and pulling your chest as far away from the space in front of you as you can; then, do the opposite, pulling your chest forward to bring your spine back to upright. Your body may tend to make the movement from the neck or the pelvis. Try to isolate it to the upper back.

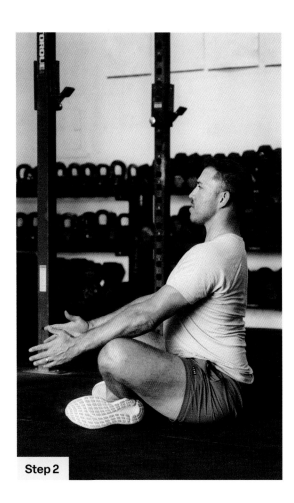

Step 2

MODIFICATIONS

Sit on a pillow, prop, or stool to build capacity for holding this upright seated position.

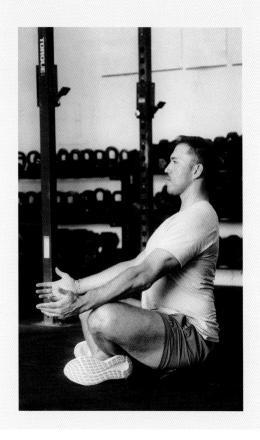

Step 2

Sit upright and hold this position for 30 seconds, or as long as you can. Remember to breathe big into the torso. After 30 seconds (or your maximum hold), relax, move your body, then get right back into it again. See if you can hold this position longer this time.

Step 3

Repeat 3 to 5 times.

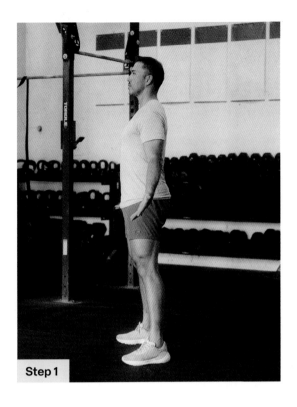

Step 1

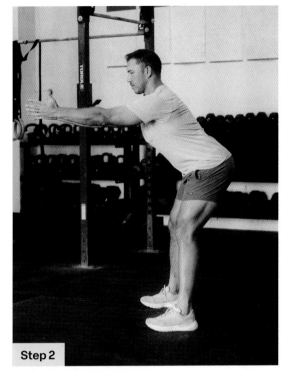

Step 2

EXERCISE 7

Hip Hinge

Mobility and strength in the hip joints are important. The hip hinge disperses force across the body's entire back side and all the muscles, tendons, and ligaments making up your posterior chain. Building trust in the hip joints translates to being confident when getting down on to and up from the floor.

Step 1

Stand tall with your feet twice as wide as hip-width apart.

Step 2

Pull your hips back into a hinge, keeping your feet strong on the floor. Try to generate 80 percent of the movement from your hips (not by arching your lower back or bending your knees). Counterweight your arms forward to try to get your hips back another inch or two (3 to 5 cm). In this position, your hips should be pulled back behind your knees, and your knees slightly behind your ankles, all while keeping a strong support base with your feet.

Step 3

When confident with steps 1 and 2, make this dynamic by flowing in and out of this hinge position. Repeat 10 to 15 times, go slowly, and match your inhales to the hinging movements and exhales to coming out of the hinge position.

MODIFICATIONS

If you don't fully trust pulling your hips back (maybe it causes lower back pain or your balance feels compromised), hold on to a table or desk in front of you for support. As you feel more confident with this movement, experiment with less reliance on the table or desk.

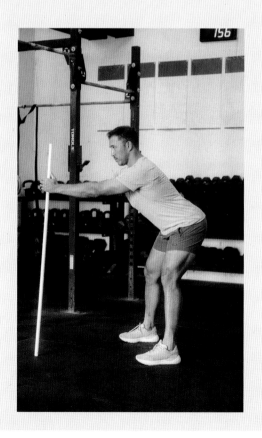

BALANCE AND CONTROL

Lower body strength and mobility are crucial for getting up off the floor; equally important is balance and control, which foster confidence, prevent falls and injuries, and allow for steady and controlled transitions from the floor to standing.

EXERCISES FOR BALANCE AND CONTROL

These next exercises will build strength, balance, and *control* in the joints and muscles that help you get up from and down on to the ground.

Where Should I Feel It?

You will feel the Isometric Lunge (page 62) on the top of the front leg, just above the knee, as it works endurance in the quadriceps muscle group. When Standing on One Foot (page 63), you'll feel your hip flexor on the bent raised leg, and in the muscles in the foot and those supporting the hip on the standing leg.

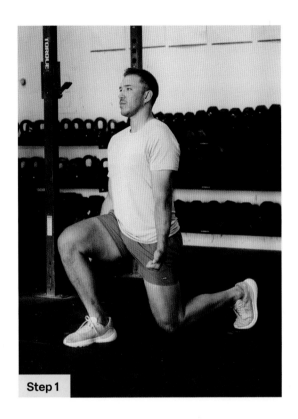

Step 1

Isometric Lunge

Knee strength and pain are concerns for many when transitioning positions. The Isometric Lunge builds stamina in the leg muscles—specifically, the quadriceps—but it also works on split stance balance.

Step 1

Place one foot in front of the other in a split stance slightly wider than hip-width apart. Drop down into a lunge so your front knee is bent to about 90 degrees and your back knee is hovering off the ground. Hold this position for 30 seconds, or as long as you are able. Return to a standing position.

Step 2

Repeat, switching the front foot in your stance.

Step 3

Repeat twice more on each side, alternating, for 3 reps total in each session.

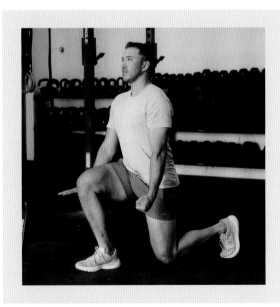

MODIFICATIONS

Hold onto a prop, like a chair or table, for support as needed.

Standing on One Foot

Being able to balance and use your muscles for support is a valuable skill. For this exercise, focus on keeping your pelvis stacked over your hips.

Step 1

Stand on one foot and march the other foot up so the knee is bent at 90 degrees, at hip height. Keep the hip of the standing leg actively pulled under the pelvis, not kicking out to the side. Hold this position for 30 seconds, or as long as you are able. Return to a standing position.

Step 2

Repeat on the other side, switching your standing foot.

Step 3

Repeat twice more on each side, alternating, for 3 reps total in each session.

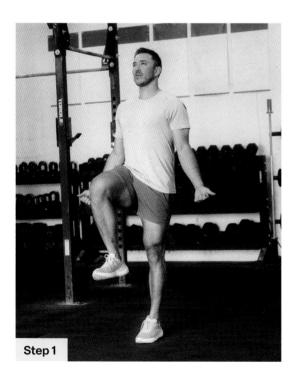

Step 1

MODIFICATIONS

If your balance feels unstable, use a table or wall for support. To increase the challenge, add a component of instability: Stand on a foam pad or a folded towel.

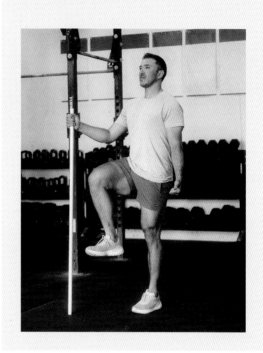

CHECKING IN

Practice these exercises for 4 to 6 weeks, then reflect and re-assess. You can attempt the self-assessment (see page 47) any time and compare notes to gauge progress. Remember, this work can take time. Be patient with yourself! You are building the strength, mobility, and control required to get up off the floor independently.

CHAPTER 7

REACH OVERHEAD

"Can someone help me with this bag? I'm too old to lift it,"
I heard a woman ask as I boarded a flight. I volunteered to help, and as I proceeded to my seat I thought, *She can't be more than fifty, yet she's convinced she's too old.*
Too old to invest in herself, too old to be independent—too old to lift her bag.

As we age, physiological changes occur that do make building strength and staying active more challenging. Reaching overhead is a fundamental everyday movement that requires strength, mobility, and control.

Try This: Overhead Carry Test

Perform a light warm-up, such as shoulder rolls, arm circles, or other dynamic stretches, to prepare your muscles, and set a distance or time standard for the test; I suggest 20 seconds or 20 feet (6 m) with each arm. Choose a space where you can walk freely without obstructions; select a weight you can hold overhead comfortably.

1. Standing with feet shoulder-width apart, hold the weight in one hand. Press it overhead until your arm is fully extended, with your biceps close to your ear. Engage your core, with back straight, shoulders level.
2. Walk forward slowly, maintaining the weight overhead. Keep your posture upright; avoid leaning to one side or arching your back. Maintain a steady, controlled gait for a set distance or time.
3. Switch the weight to the other hand and repeat.

Assess

- *Strength* : For each arm, record the distance or time the weight is held overhead without experiencing fatigue or loss of form.

Note Bring awareness to core control and keep your rib cage stacked over your pelvis as you reach. This ensures that the shoulders and upper back are challenged rather than the lower back, which we can tend to arch when reaching overhead. Modify the movements as needed—it is better to do a movement with modification than to compromise your safety.

- *Mobility and comfort*:
  - ▸ Compare range of motion and ability to get your arms overhead on both sides.
  - ▸ Is there discomfort or pain in your shoulders, neck, or upper back during the movement? Seek professional guidance if you experience significant pain or discomfort.
- *Balance and control* : Did you feel strong and stable? Note any wobbling or difficulty maintaining the weight overhead in a steady position. Check that your arm remains fully extended with your biceps close to your ear.

If you can walk with the weight overhead, maintaining proper form and without pain, you likely have good shoulder strength, mobility, balance, and control for overhead movements. Try a heavier weight or increase the time or distance assessed.

STRENGTH

To increase capacity while reaching overhead, there are two important things to focus on: building strength getting the object from the floor to your chest in a secure position and building strength in the pressing movement—getting the object away from your chest and above your head.

Safety First If you have an injury or medical condition—especially with the shoulders, neck, or upper back—consult your health care provider before undertaking these exercises.

EXERCISES FOR STRENGTH

Overhead lifting primarily engages the shoulders, upper back, and arm muscles, which must be strong to stabilize and control what is being lifted and to reduce the risk of injury. When lifting overhead, the body must generate sufficient force to press up, which is why the core and spine muscles are also important. This combination of strength and stability makes the movement more effective and ensures that everyday tasks and activities can be performed safely and confidently.

Where Should I Feel It?

The Kettlebell Clean (page 66) engages your legs, core, and upper body. The Overhead Press (page 68) uses the muscles that support the shoulder joints and spine—if you feel it in the lower back, don't overarch as you press. Keep the movement isolated to the shoulders.

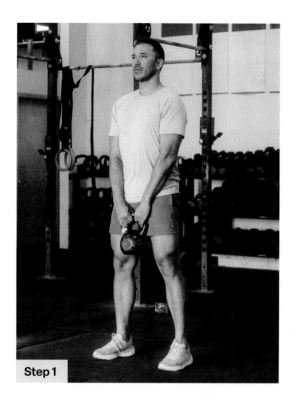

Step 1

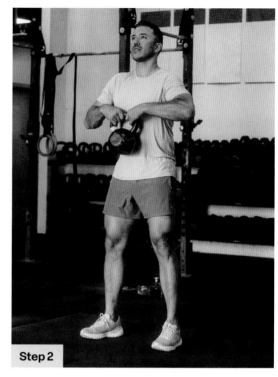

Step 2

EXERCISE 1

Kettlebell Clean

There are many ways to lift an object to a position (up to your chest) that prepares you to press it overhead. I like the Kettlebell Clean to train for this because the kettlebell's design makes it easy to keep the weight close to your center of gravity, which is important for safety and strength. Use a weight based on your current strength, capacity, and goals: A beginner should use a lighter weight, 10 to 20 pounds (4.5 to 9 kg); someone more experienced can use something heavier, 20 to 55+ pounds (9 to 25+ kg).

Step 1

Stand with feet hip-width apart. Place a kettlebell between your feet. Unlock your knees and hinge your hips back, bend at the waist, and grab the bell's handle with both hands using an overhand grip, keeping your arms straight down.

Step 2

Drive through your heels to stand up—much of the power comes from the legs—lifting the kettlebell up to your waist. Keep the kettlebell close to your body with arms straight.

Step 3

As you continue to raise the kettlebell past waist height, your elbows will bend as you prepare for the clean. Pull your elbows close to your body and guide the kettlebell up toward your chest

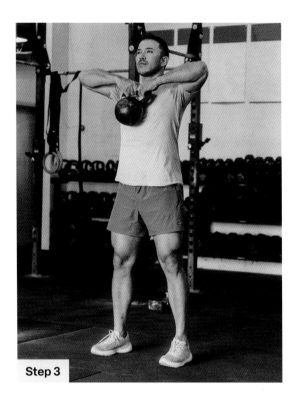

Step 3

MODIFICATIONS

- No matter your capacity, start with a manageable weight until you feel confident with the movement's mechanics.
- Lift from an elevated surface: Place the weight on a short bench or box instead of the floor.
- Segment the movement. Master the "high pull" (steps 1 and 2). Set up the kettlebell the same way, but instead of transitioning your grip to the horns and completing the clean (step 3), drive your elbows wide and pull the kettlebell high up your torso, then bring the weight back to the starting position with control.

while simultaneously switching your grip: Rotate your wrists (keep the bottom of the kettlebell facing down) and slide your hands to grip the kettlebell by the horns (the sides of the handle). Your elbows should point down and the kettlebell should rest against your chest.

Step 4

To complete the repetition, follow the path back to the floor: Return your hands to the overhand grip. Keep the kettlebell close to your body as you hinge your hips back at the waist and lower the weight to the floor between your feet. Repeat 8 to 10 times.

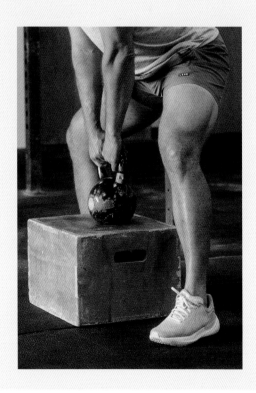

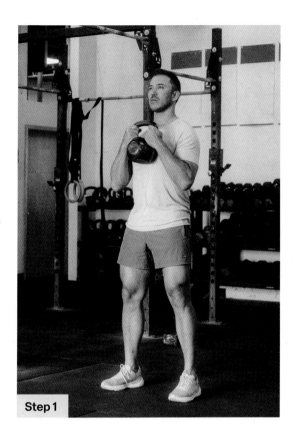

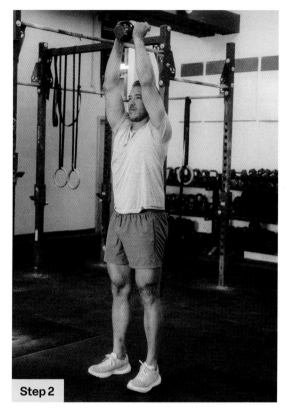

EXERCISE 2

Overhead Press

With the weight securely in position to move it up overhead (exercise 1, Kettlebell Clean, page 66), we now need to work on generating the arm, shoulder, and core strength to press the weight up and overhead.

Step 1

Stand with your feet about hip-width apart and create a solid base connection between your feet and the floor. Hold the weight securely at your chest.

Step 2

Check your core: Keep your rib cage stacked over your hips. Your spine may tend to arch as you press up and overhead, finding more movement in the lower back rather than the upper back or shoulders where we want it, which can be uncomfortable.

Step 3

Press the weight up and overhead, straightening your elbows as you do.

Step 4

Safely bring the weight back to your chest to complete the repetition. Perform 8 to 10 reps.

MOBILITY

We now have tools to build strength in the upper body and core to help lift and press overhead. However, it can be difficult to perform these tasks efficiently without adequate mobility in the shoulder joints and upper back. We spend significant portions of our days flexed forward, over our phone, our workstation, sitting in chairs, in cars, repeatedly in the same positions—which are not inherently "bad," but can make us complacent, forgetting the value of exposing our body to other ranges of motion.

EXERCISES FOR MOBILITY

These exercises target the shoulders and upper back to cultivate the mobility necessary to press overhead.

Where Should I Feel It?

You'll feel these exercises in the upper back joints and the muscles that support the shoulder joints. The sensation in the upper back should feel like pressure, not a pinching or sharp sensation; if it does, stop and try the modifications.

EXERCISE 3

Arms Up the Wall Lift-Offs

This movement helps with flexion through the shoulder joint, which is critical for lifting overhead.

Step 1

Stand 6 to 12 inches (15 to 30 cm) from a wall, facing the wall; your feet should be hip-width apart and your rib cage stacked over your pelvis. Avoid arching your lower back more than what your standing posture allows. Bring your arms overhead, make two fists, and place the pinky side of your fists against the wall. Keep your neck tall.

Step 2

Check neck, spine, and hip alignment and generate stiffness throughout the entire body to prepare to isolate movement to the shoulder joint. Lift your fists 3 to 5 inches (7.5 to 12.5 cm) from the wall—both at once, or one at a time. Hold this position for 7 to 10 seconds. Return your fists to the wall. Repeat 6 to 8 times on both sides.

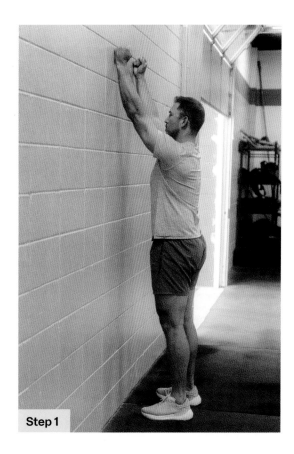

Step 1

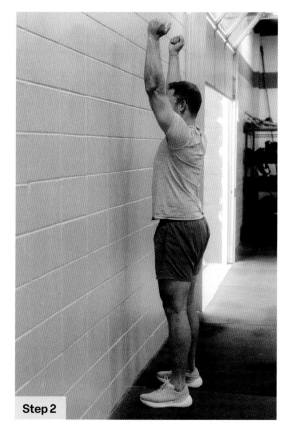

Step 2

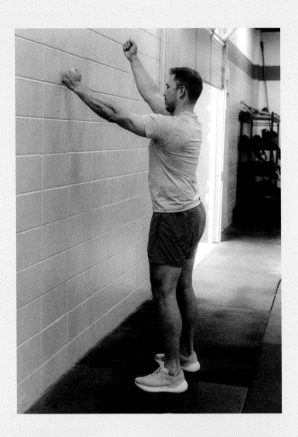

MODIFICATION 1

If you're moving the neck, lower back, knees, or other area, your shoulders may not be conditioned for the range of motion being asked of them. Walk your feet away from the wall, creating more space, with your arms up at an angle.

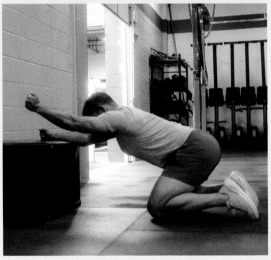

MODIFICATION 2

To advance the exercise, use gravity to create resistance. Being parallel to the floor forces isolation of movement to the shoulder joint. Kneel in front of a bench or table and lift your arms directly away from the bench and, therefore, the floor (instead of perpendicular to the floor as in the original exercise).

Back to the Wall Press

This exercise addresses the upper back, which has a natural forward curve (flexed) but also the capacity to extend—a range of motion we don't expose it to often—and create space for the shoulder joints to reach overhead.

Step 1

Place a stool against a wall and take a seat, facing away from the wall. Bend your elbows at 90 degrees, out to the sides like goal posts, and bring both arms against the wall. The back of your head, your shoulder blades, elbows, and the backs of your wrists and hands should touch the wall, too.

Step 2

Slide the backs of your arms up the wall while maintaining all points of contact noted in step 1. You might feel pressure, or a "challenge," at the base of your neck, down to the space between your shoulder blades. This is your upper back extending.

Step 3

Bring your elbows down and return to the starting position while keeping the points of contact with the wall noted in step 1. Repeat 6 to 8 times.

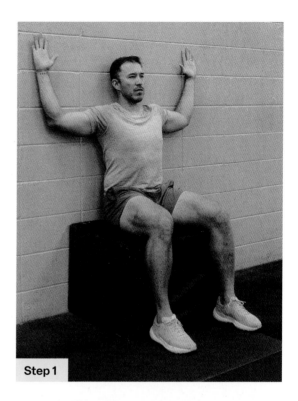

Step 1

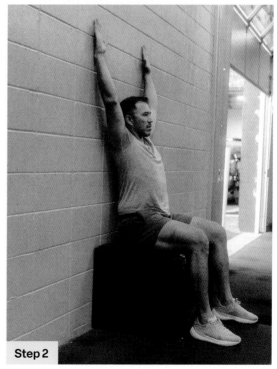

Step 2

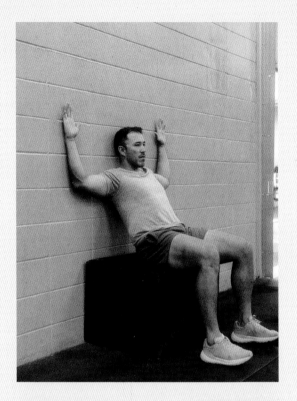

MODIFICATION 1

If this feels challenging, scoot your seat away from the wall, creating more of an angle for your arms to rest on the wall—start with 12 inches (30 cm) from the wall. As you can perform the exercise with more ease, bring your seat closer to the wall, 1 inch (2.5 cm) at a time. This will put less focus on the upper back.

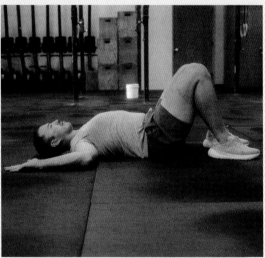

MODIFICATION 2

Or, lie on your back, with knees bent and feet on the floor.

EXERCISE 5

Forward Single-Arm Wall Walks

The ability to reach overhead into flexion supports activities like lifting something overhead or climbing/pulling from an overhead position. The Forward Single-Arm Wall Walk builds capacity for overhead movements, but with the safety of the wall. As you repeat the exercise, note any changes you feel.

Step 1

Stand facing a wall, 16 to 24 inches (40 to 60 cm) away, feet hip-width apart. Reach your right hand to the wall at shoulder height.

Step 2

Keep your entire torso still. Isolating the movement to the shoulder, slowly walk your fingers up the wall. As you do so, your elbow extends, and your hand will reach up the wall overhead in front of you. Keep crawling up until your arm is straight and your elbow is completely extended. Walk your hand down to the starting point. Repeat 8 to 10 times.

Step 3

Switch to the other side and repeat 8 to 10 times.

MODIFICATIONS

If this feels challenging, start by standing farther away from the wall, 18 to 30 inches (45 to 75 cm), so when your elbow is fully extended, your hand isn't as far up the wall.

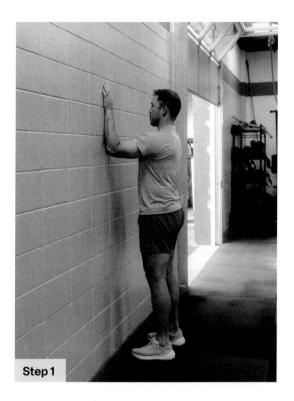

Step 1

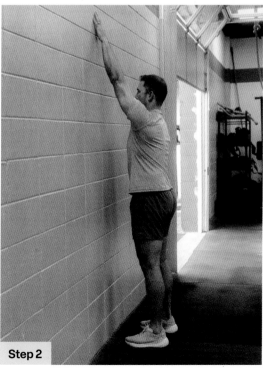

Step 2

BALANCE AND CONTROL

The shoulder joint, one of the largest and most mobile joints in the body, requires a greater spectrum of mobility and stability to function properly. Proper joint control helps stabilize the shoulder girdle, allowing the muscles to work efficiently and reducing the risk of dislocations, impingements, or other injuries. Additionally, balanced shoulder function supports the scapula (shoulder blade) in providing a stable base for arm movement, facilitating smooth and coordinated lifting motions, allowing you to perform overhead tasks—whether lifting heavy objects, stretching to reach high places, or lifting weights—more confidently.

EXERCISES FOR BALANCE AND CONTROL

Here I explore movement to build strength, balance, and control in the ball-and-socket joint, as well as the scapulothoracic joint of the shoulder girdle, essential for reaching overhead with confidence and ease.

Where Should I Feel It?

The movements when reaching overhead primarily work the muscles in the shoulder girdle, as well as the core. To isolate the area we are working on—in this case, the shoulder—the neighboring muscles must work hard to create tension or stiffen up.

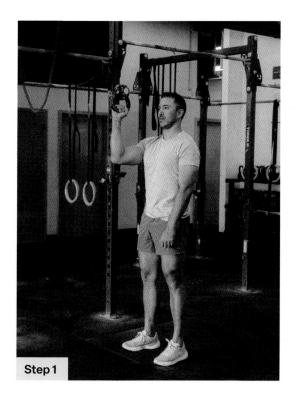

Step 1

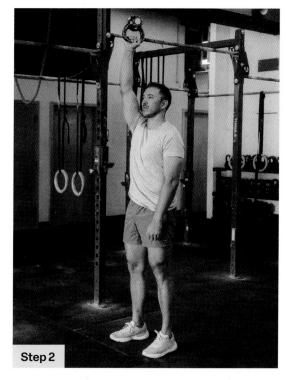

Step 2

EXERCISE 6

Bottoms-Up Kettlebell Press

The unstable nature of the inverted kettlebell in this exercise forces the shoulder muscles to work hard to maintain balance, which enhances proprioception (awareness of joint position), strengthens the smaller stabilizing muscles, and improves overall shoulder joint control.

Step 1

Stand solidly, feet hip-width apart. Place a lightweight kettlebell between your feet. With both hands, lift the kettlebell to shoulder height (see exercise 1, Kettlebell Clean, page 66). Transition the kettlebell to one hand and carefully invert the bell, holding the handle facing the floor and the bell facing the ceiling.

Step 2

When ready to press, bring awareness to your core and stiffen the entire body to help isolate movement to the shoulder. Slowly press the kettlebell upward, extending the elbow of the pressing arm fully. Focus on maintaining the kettlebell's inverted position—keep a steady pace to avoid excessive wobbling.

Step 3

With the bell overhead, slowly, with control, bend the elbow and come back to the starting position (step 1). Perform 6 to 8 reps on this side.

Step 4

Repeat on the other side.

MODIFICATION

If this movement is new, get used to holding the kettlebell inverted without pressing it overhead. Do this by repeating step 1. Advance the movement by bringing your elbow up to shoulder height, so your arm is bent at 90 degrees, and work on holding the kettlebell still in this position.

CHECKING IN

Take 4 to 6 weeks with these movements before repeating the Overhead Carry Test (page 64). Compare the notes you took during the initial test to gauge objective and subjective progress. To progress, you do need to advance or, in some instances, increase the weight used; however, it is important not to rush. Reaching overhead can be a complex and challenging skill to maintain.

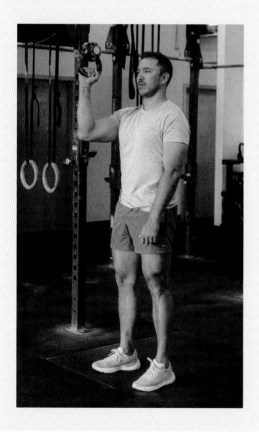

CHAPTER 8

CARRY AND TRANSPORT

"I just want to be able to pick up my granddaughter and carry her to her crib."

When we think about the hallmarks of a long, healthy life, we envision robust physical strength, mobility, independence, and the ability to perform everyday tasks with ease. One underrated yet profoundly important measure of this is the ability to lift things and transport them. In training, we call this the farmer's carry.

The farmer's carry is straightforward: You lift heavy weights and walk a certain distance. Despite its simplicity, this exercise engages multiple muscle groups—from grip strength in the hands to the muscles in your shoulders, back, core, and legs. It's a full-body workout that builds muscle while enhancing coordination, balance, and stability.

Moreover, farmer's carries enhance proprioception, the body's ability to sense its position in space. This heightened awareness is crucial for balance and coordination, reducing the likelihood of falls and improving overall mobility. For older adults, maintaining a strong sense of balance can be the difference between independence and reliance on others for daily activities.

Grip strength is an area of physical health I am passionate about when it comes to aging stronger. And the benefit is, that most people see results in almost all other areas of strength as a result of the exercises here.

Note Most modifications add or subtract weight from the movement. Choose weights you feel confident lifting and supporting as you move.

Try This: Grip Hold Test

Warm up the core and upper body with push-ups, a brisk 5-minute walk, and some upper body stretches.

1. Gather a pair of heavy dumbbells, kettlebells, or even weight plates you can hold comfortably for at least 15 seconds. Pick the heaviest weight you can lift.
2. Stand with your feet shoulder-width apart and place a heavy weight on each side of your body.
3. Bending at your knees and hips, squat down and lift the weights back to standing. Hold the weights firmly at your sides with a strong grip.
4. Stand tall with shoulders back, chest up, and rib cage stacked over your pelvis. Hold for as long as possible; if you're holding the weight for longer than 2 minutes, it's too light. Re-test with heavier weights.

Assess

- *Performance*:
  - ▸ How long did you hold the weight and how much weight did you grab? Could you maintain a strong grip the entire time without needing to rest or readjust?
  - ▸ Did you keep an upright posture without leaning to one side or arching your back?
- *Comfort* : Note any discomfort or pain in the shoulders, neck, back, or hands during the movement, and any signs of strain or fatigue in particular areas.

STRENGTH

As we age, maintaining muscle mass and functional strength becomes increasingly critical. Sarcopenia, age-related loss of muscle mass, is a common concern that can lead to a reduction in independence. Continually challenging a variety of muscles counteracts this decline and promotes growth and muscle maintenance, keeping you strong, healthy, and independent. The act of carrying weight also stimulates bone density, vital in preventing osteoporosis and reducing the risk of falls and fractures.

One compelling reason farmer's carries are invaluable for longevity is their direct application to daily life. Consider the simple act of carrying groceries from the car or subway to the kitchen. This routine chore can become a daunting task as we age without the necessary strength and stability. Farmer's carries simulate this movement, teaching our body how to distribute weight evenly, engage the core for support, and use the legs for stability, ensuring we can perform this motion efficiently and without injury.

 Safety First We want challenge without compromising safety. When picking up a weight, keep it close to your center of gravity (close to your body) and lift with your legs— bend your knees into a squat, grab the object, and lift.

EXERCISES FOR STRENGTH

The farmer's carry can be done many ways: arms down to the side, arms overhead, mixed grip, or really any way you can think of—there is no right, wrong, better, or worse way to do it. We will test a few variations to build strength. The limiting factor is typically grip strength, so choose a weight you can pick up and put down safely: If you're a beginner, start with 10 to 25 pounds (4.5 to 11 kg); if you're more advanced, grab something heavier—30 to 70+ pounds (14 to 32+ kg).

Where Should I Feel It?

You will feel these movements in your hands, forearms, and shoulders, as well as through your core and into your hips.

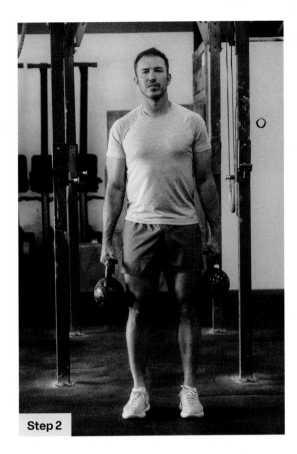

Step 2

EXERCISE 1

Suitcase Carry

Building capacity in this activity is simple . . . progress your carries. Do more carries, add weight, or carry for longer distances. The Suitcase Carry can be done with free weights, household objects such as bags, buckets, and water jugs, or anything with a handle.

Step 1

Choose a distance you can complete easily, say 25 to 30 feet (7.5 to 9 m).

Step 2

Stand with feet about hip-width apart. Position your "suitcases" one to each side, with your arms straight down at your sides. Keeping your shoulder blades actively pulled down and away from your neck, bend your knees into a squat, pick up both weights, and return to a standing position.

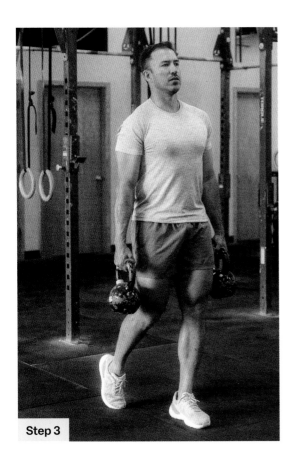
Step 3

MODIFICATIONS

If your chosen distance is too difficult to complete, decrease your weight or distance. If it's too easy, increase the weight or distance.

Step 3

Keep your arms down to the sides, maintain space between your rib cage and pelvis, and walk forward. The heavier the load, the more your body will tend to pull down toward the ground. Think about fighting up and away from gravity, keeping your body tall and strong. When you reach your chosen spot, turn around and return to where you started.

Step 4

Put down the weights, rest for 60 seconds, and repeat.

EXERCISE 2

Racked Carry

This farmer's carry variation requires the weight to be held up at the shoulders. Choose a lighter weight than you used in exercise 1, Suitcase Carry (page 80).

Step 1

Keeping the weight close to your body, lift it to your shoulders—either on top of or in front of the shoulders. It's easy to dump into your lower back, so keep your rib cage stacked over your pelvis. Note that arching your lower back is not a dangerous posture; it's a normal range of motion. However, the goal is to absorb the weight using muscles, not joints. Excessive arching in your back can result in the small joints in the lower back taking on that additional force instead of the muscles and might cause discomfort over time.

Step 2

With the weight in a secure position, walk forward 25 to 30 feet (7.5 to 9 m). Walk back to your starting position.

Step 3

Put down the weight, rest for 60 seconds, and repeat.

MODIFICATIONS

Adjust the weight and distance depending on your capacity and goals. You can also build endurance just by holding the weight in the racked position (step 1) without walking.

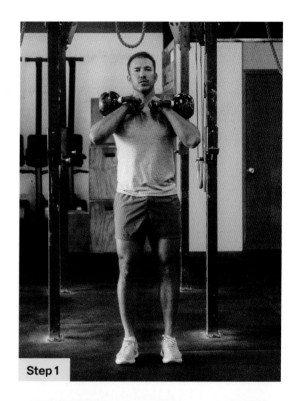

Step 1

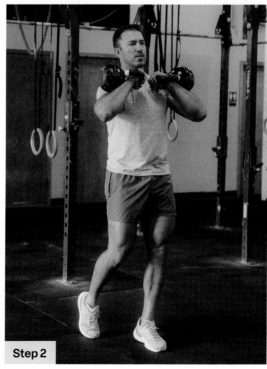

Step 2

EXERCISE 3

Single-Arm Racked Carry

This exercise combines the movements from exercises 1 (Suitcase Carry, page 80) and 2 (Racked Carry, page 82): one arm in a suitcase hold, the other in a racked position. Choose a lighter weight for the Racked Carry and a heavier weight for the Suitcase Carry.

Step 1

Bring the lighter weight up to your shoulders in the racked position (see exercise 2, Racked Carry) and hold the other down to your side in a suitcase position (see exercise 1, Suitcase Carry).

Step 2

Walk forward 25 to 30 feet (7.5 to 9 m). Note the different challenges on each side and try to walk in a straight line without leaning to either side. When you get to the end, drop the weights, switch your grip, and walk back to where you started.

Step 3

Put down the weights, rest for 60 seconds, and repeat.

MODIFICATIONS

Adjust the weight and distance depending on your capacity and goals. If this mixed grip feels too advanced, repeat exercises 1 (Suitcase Carry) and 2 (Racked Carry) for now.

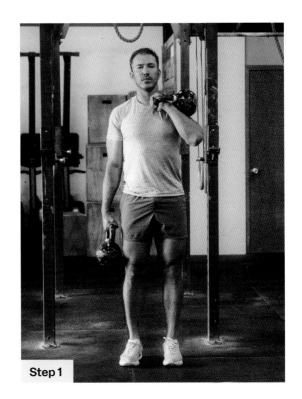

Step 1

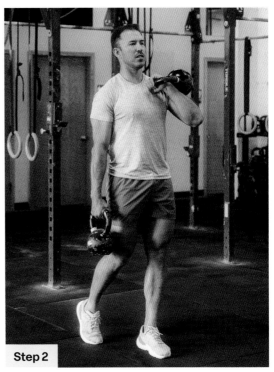

Step 2

EXERCISE 4

Tennis Ball Squeeze

Squeezing a ball might not seem like an exercise, but it works the small muscles in the wrist, hand, and fingers to build grip endurance. You can also use a rolled-up towel or pair of socks, or a stress ball.

Step 1

Hold the ball with your dominant hand, elbow bent at 90 degrees in front of you, forearm parallel to the ground.

Step 2

Squeeze the ball with only your fingers— don't use your thumb. Hold for 5 to 7 seconds. Repeat 8 to 10 times.

Step 3

Repeat with your nondominant hand.

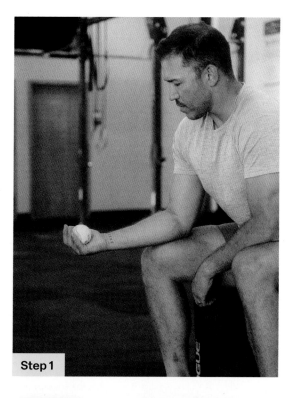

Step 1

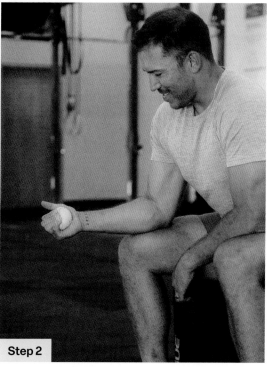

Step 2

MODIFICATIONS

Adjust how long you squeeze, or the firmness of the object—squeezing a pair of socks for 10 seconds is easier than squeezing a lacrosse ball.

MOBILITY

Mobility may not seem critical for something like a carry, but adding range of motion focus to the upper back and shoulders can ensure optimal load distribution—essential for preventing injuries and maximizing efficiency. Good mobility in these areas complements a strong, stable shoulder girdle, supporting the weight being carried and reducing strain on the lower back. Improved load distribution also enables you to carry heavier loads more comfortably and for longer distances.

EXERCISES FOR MOBILITY

The following exercises mobilize the upper back and shoulder joint to set up the carry for success.

Where Should I Feel It?

The Internal and External Rotation Wring Out (page 86) targets the shoulder joint at the ball and socket. You might also feel a stretch down the biceps, into the forearm and wrist. The thoracic rotation targets the upper back and rib cage. You should feel a deep stretch between the shoulder blades and along the sides of the body. If pinching or sharp pain occurs, back off the range of motion and slow the movements.

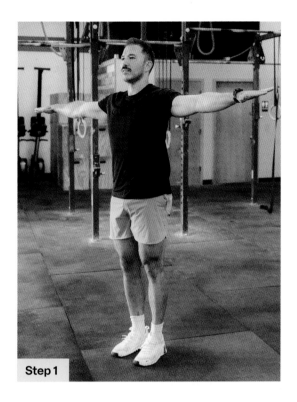

Step 1

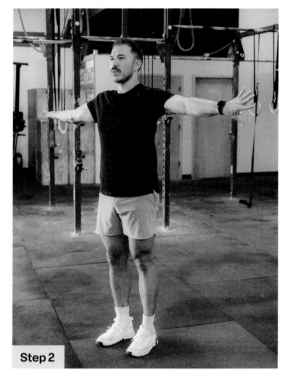

Step 2

EXERCISE 5

Internal and External Rotation Wring Out

Having internal and external rotation in the shoulder joint is important when holding objects and carrying them. This exercise actively builds range of motion while bringing awareness to the shoulder blades and core muscles.

Step 1

Stand with feet about hip-width apart. Bring both arms straight out to the side creating a *T* with your arms and body.

Step 2

Drive tension into the floor and up through the leg and torso muscles to stabilize and create a solid base to move from. Bring focus to the shoulder joint and rotate one shoulder forward and one backward. It is easy to perform the movement though the forearms, so work to initiate movement from the shoulder. Imagine wringing out a towel. Repeat, rotating your shoulders the opposite way.

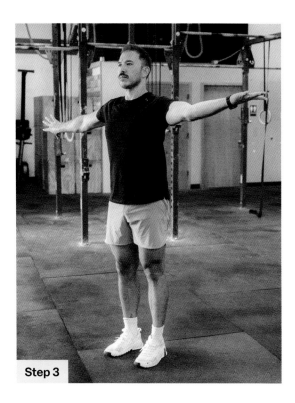

Step 3

Step 3

Alternate the directions you do this for 8 to 10 reps total.

MODIFICATIONS

If you have difficulty rotating both arms at the same time, isolate one side: Lie on your right side (on the floor or a bed). Reach the top arm up to the sky and rotate it from the shoulder joint clockwise, then counterclockwise. Repeat on the other side.

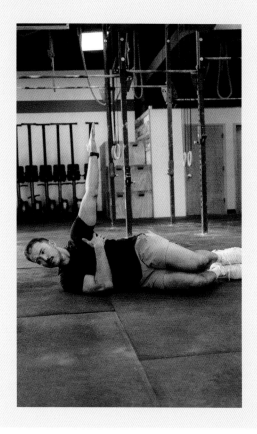

EXERCISE 6

Kneeling Thoracic Rotation

Another area of mobility focus is the thoracic spine (from the neck to the bottom of the ribs) and rib cage. While walking, there is a lot of subtle rotation in this area, so maintaining strength and mobility here is valuable. For the exercise, it's important to build central tension by holding on to a prop, like a ball, cushion, or rolled-up blanket.

Step 1

Assume a kneeling position (see Reverse Lunge with Reach, page 48), with both bent knees on the floor hug your prop (see modifications) against your chest.

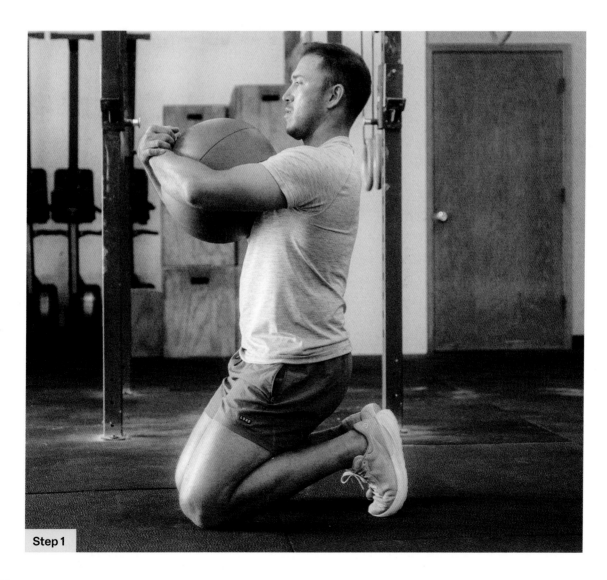

Step 1

Step 2

From center, rotate your upper body toward the side of your planted foot as far as you can, getting as much pain-free rotation in the upper back as you can. Hold for 1 second. Come back to center. Repeat 8 to 10 times on this side.

Step 3

Switch your foot position in the kneeling position and rotate toward the other side. Repeat 8 to 10 times on this side.

MODIFICATIONS

If you don't have a prop, cross one hand over to the opposite shoulder, then the other, stacking your arms over each other as if giving yourself a tight hug. This also creates the central tension needed to access more rotation in the upper back.

If it is uncomfortable to get into a kneeling position, place a pillow or a pad under your knees on the ground.

Step 2

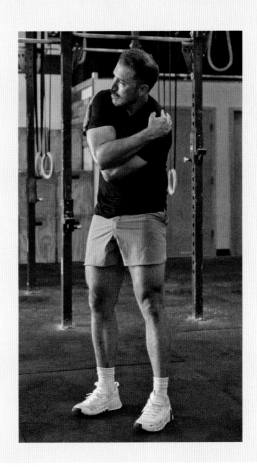

BALANCE AND CONTROL

Balance and control are crucial for carrying heavy objects, especially awkward ones. Distributing weight evenly across your body allows for a larger, more confident base of support to carry from. We can do this by improving balance and learning how to isolate movements in the spine and hips. Good balance lets you navigate various terrains and obstacles without losing stability—essential for avoiding trips, slips, and falls. Joint control helps us handle the object securely, adjusting as needed to keep stable and prevent slipping or dropping. This is particularly important in dynamic environments where sudden changes in direction or unexpected movements might occur.

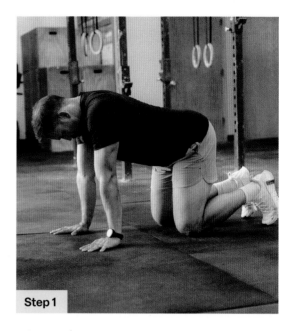
Step 1

EXERCISES FOR BALANCE AND CONTROL

Building spinal control and endurance on one leg cultivates a solid foundation for a strong carry. Well-controlled joints provide support during movement, especially when lifting heavy objects and transporting them across long distances.

EXERCISE 7

Segmented Cat-Cow

Finding control in the small joints of the spine helps distribute force when carrying heavy objects. It is typically easier to do in a quadruped position (on your hands and knees in a tabletop position), when your body is parallel to the floor. Go slowly—isolating each individual vertebra is challenging. Give yourself grace and respect that, for most people, this is a work in progress.

Where Should I Feel It?

You'll feel the Segmented Cat-Cow (above) in the spine—the better you get at isolating the movement, the more you will feel it. The Hip Clock (page 92) challenges single-leg balance, which you will feel primarily in the muscles supporting the hip joint—from the glutes to the adductors (inner thighs) to the hamstrings.

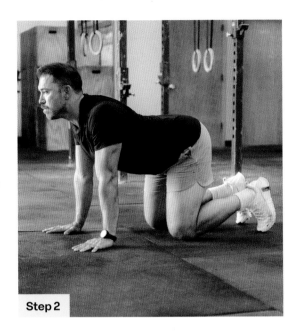

Step 2

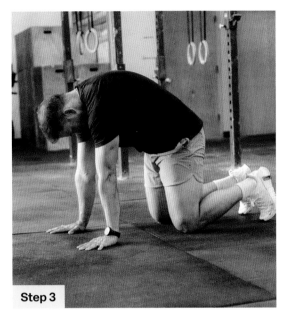

Step 3

Step 1

Get into a quadruped position on the floor, hands directly under your shoulders, shoulder-width apart, fingertips forward, knees directly under your hips, hip-width apart.

Step 2

Starting with "cow," inhale deeply and lift your sit bones upward, tilting your pelvis up. One vertebra at a time, pull your spine down toward the floor (into extension) like a wave until you reach your neck, then lift your head and gaze straight ahead. Your spine will be sagging toward the ground.

Step 3

Move into "cat" pose. Start by tucking your chin under and, like a wave, round your spine one vertebra at a time—from the neck to the upper back to the lower back, and finally, to the pelvis— into flexion. Your spine will be arching up away from the ground.

Step 4

Repeat steps 1 through 3, 4 to 6 times.

MODIFICATIONS

Relax your focus on "segmenting" and simply get the spine into its end ranges of motion. This is further discussed in chapter 11 (page 124).

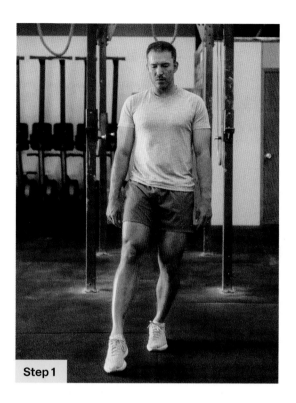

Step 1

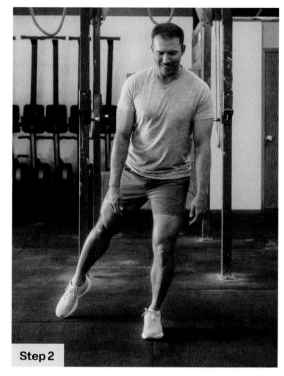

Step 2

EXERCISE 8

Hip Clock

This exercise challenges the lower body, specifically the muscles that support the hip joint. Being on one foot in any capacity integrates all the muscles from the foot to the pelvis. Performing unilateral work not only improves balance but also strength and proprioception.

Step 1

Stand tall on your left foot. Keep your torso upright; do not lock the left knee. Keeping 95 percent of your weight on your left foot, with your right toes, gently tap the one o'clock position on the floor.

Step 2

Return to the starting position, but now tap your right toes back and to the right to the four o'clock position on the floor.

Step 3

Return to the starting position. The third tap is the eight o'clock position: Pull your right foot behind your left leg. Tap back and to the left with your right toes, mimicking the movement pattern of a curtsy lunge.

Step 4

Repeat on the other side, standing on the right foot and tapping with the left foot to the eleven o'clock, eight o'clock, and four o'clock positions.

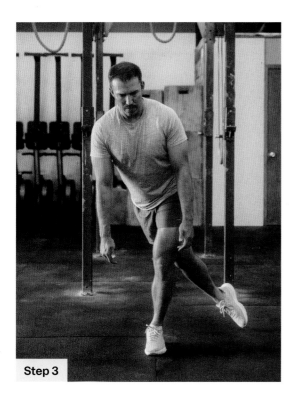

Step 3

CHECKING IN

This chapter is all about grip strength and teaching your body to move independently. The Grip Hold Test (page 79) also acts as a strength and endurance builder. Incorporating the targeted strength, mobility, balance, and control exercises enhances your grip strength, core stability, and overall endurance, making carrying and transporting heavy items safer and more effective. Keep at it and watch your capacity grow!

MODIFICATIONS

Using a countertop or a walking stick to assist with balance builds capacity in these movements. Use as little support as possible so the hip, leg, and foot are forced to work. As the movement becomes easier, use less support.

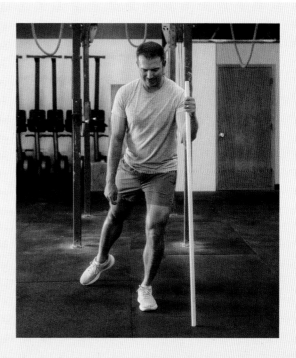

CHAPTER 9

PICK UP OFF THE GROUND

"I can't lift that; I had a disk injury and bending over makes it worse."

I hear this frequently, and while there are situations when avoiding movements can be a good short-term recovery strategy, the human body is highly adaptable, with the capacity to change, grow, and heal—as long as we put it in the proper environments to do so.

As we age, being able to continue to lift things off the ground is crucial. It directly impacts our functional independence and quality of life. Maintaining mobility and strength becomes increasingly important to perform daily activities like picking things up around the house, carrying items from the car, or moving heavier objects around the yard safely and efficiently. The more we expose ourselves to everyday movements that are part of life, like bending over to put on socks or lifting a box off the ground, the more conditioned our body becomes for these activities. And enhanced hip, knee, and ankle health improves overall balance and stability, vital for preventing falls and injuries.

Try This: Touch Your Toes

This simple assessment evaluates mobility and strength, particularly in the hamstrings, lower back, and hips, and can help identify tightness, range of motion limitations, and overall flexibility. Spend a few minutes warming up, such as marching in place, doing some Segmented Cat-Cows (page 90), or walking, to prepare your muscles and joints.

1. Stand with feet hip-width apart, arms relaxed by your sides. Keep your knees straight but not locked.

Note When training to pick things up off the ground, start with lighter objects at a shorter range of motion from a raised surface like a bench or a chair. Building confidence and strength, you can progress to lifting heavier objects from lower surfaces.

2. Slowly bend forward at the hips, reaching your hands toward your toes. Keep your back as straight as possible initially, then allow it to round naturally as you reach farther. Reach as far as you can comfortably without forcing the movement.

3. Touch your toes or reach as close to them as possible. Hold this position for a few seconds.

4. Slowly return to a standing position by reversing the movements, keeping them controlled.

Assess

- How far can you reach? Can you touch your toes? Ankles? Shins? Knees?
- Does your back stay straight or round significantly? Does the spine movement feel natural and smooth?
- Keep your knees straight but not locked.
- Was there any discomfort or pain in your lower back, hamstrings, or other areas?
- Work on the exercises in this chapter and perform this assessment regularly, such as once a week, to monitor progress. Record your reached distance and any changes in comfort or flexibility.

STRENGTH

We will use the same principles for building strength to pick things up off the floor as in previous chapters for other activities, dissecting the movement and finding ways to move that feel approachable, build confidence, and develop capacity.

When building strength to lift items off the ground, most of the power comes from conditioning the leg muscles. The best way to do this is to keep the object you are lifting close to your body, under your center of gravity, rather than out in front of you. In this way, you build strength in the leg muscles rather than putting all of the demand on the spine.

Practicing these exercises gradually increases your ability to handle the everyday demands of bending and lifting, promoting joint health and flexibility. By regularly putting your joints through their full range of motion in a controlled manner, you expose them to their outer limits, thereby preserving joint integrity over time.

 Safety First If you have an injury or medical condition—especially with the lower back or hips—consult your health care provider before undertaking these exercises.

EXERCISES FOR STRENGTH

These strength exercises ensure we can continue to perform essential tasks independently, such as caring for an aging relative, engaging in hobbies, or helping a friend move, thus preserving our autonomy and enhancing our overall well-being as we age.

Where Should I Feel It?

You should feel these movements primarily in the backs of your legs, on the outside of your hips, and in the inner thighs. You will also feel some activation along the muscles around your spine. Remember, feeling this area "work" is expected—pinching or sharp pain is not.

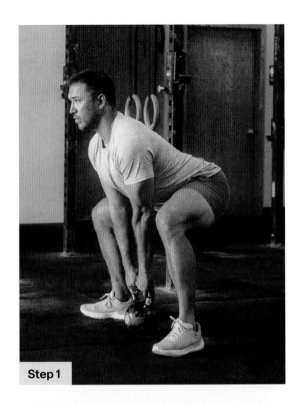

Step 1

EXERCISE 1

Sumo Squat

The Sumo Squat, compared to a traditional squat, is set up with the legs a little farther apart and the hips externally rotated (toes pointed out). This wider base of support provides more stability when lifting objects and requires strength throughout the glutes, hamstrings, and adductor muscles. It also allows you to keep a more upright torso position, which helps evenly distribute the weight being lifted throughout the spine.

Step 1

Stand with feet slightly wider than shoulder and hip-width apart and turn your toes out at about a 45-degree angle. Place a kettlebell or other heavy object (dumbbell, loaded backpack, sack of flour) between your feet. Keep the torso upright and feet planted, then squat down, driving your knees over your toes.

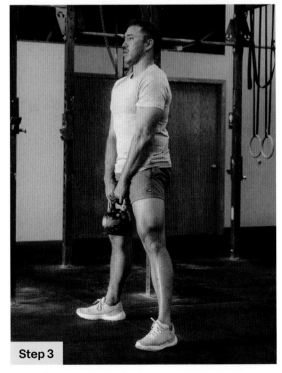

Step 3

Step 2

Grab the kettlebell handle and create some torque as if trying to break the handle in half away from you, pressing more into the pinkie side of your hands. You will feel the muscles engage on the backs of your shoulders and down the rib cage. If you aren't using a kettlebell, focus on creating tension in the object you are picking up.

Step 3

Keep the weight between your feet and drive pressure into the floor to stand up, lifting the kettlebell with you.

Step 4

Repeat 8 to 10 times.

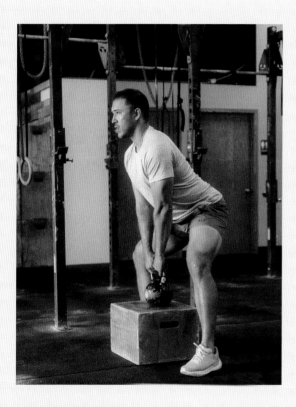

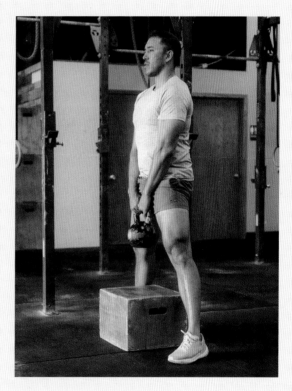

MODIFICATION 1

If it feels challenging to bend over and grab heavier objects from the floor, place the object on a prop, like a yoga block, book, or short box, to decrease the range of motion. As you build capacity, decrease the prop's height.

MODIFICATION 2

Also, widen your stance and turn out your toes a little more. This both shortens the distance between you and the floor and lets you keep your body more upright while lifting.

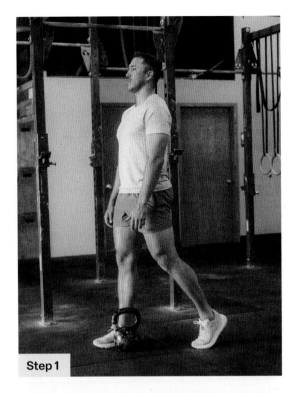

Step 1

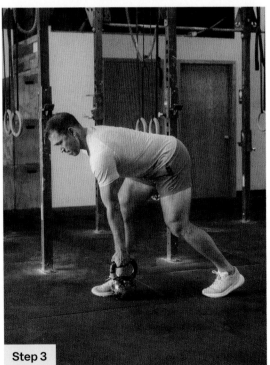

Step 3

EXERCISE 2

Single-Leg Deadlift

When we pick things up, it's common to bend over from a split stance position rather than having both feet perfectly straddled over the object being lifted. For that reason, it is valuable to condition the body for this movement. The Single-Leg Deadlift is a strength movement requiring a great deal of balance and control in the hips. It challenges the posterior chain and gets the core involved in picking things up off the ground.

Step 1

Stand with hips shoulder-width apart and place a kettlebell between your feet. Step one foot backward, keeping the other foot in its original position, leaving you in a split stance. The kettlebell should be on the ground, inside your front foot.

Step 2

Unlock your front knee and hinge your hips back, keeping most of your weight in the back of the front leg. The movement is initiated by the hip hinge, not by bending your knee and "squatting down" to grab the weight.

Step 3

Grab the weight with the hand opposite your front foot and drive your front foot into the ground to lift the weight off the floor with a straight arm until your torso is upright. The front leg does most of the work, with the back leg used more as a "kickstand."

Step 4

Return the weight to the ground, next to the inside of your front foot, following the same path you picked it up with. Initiate this movement by hinging your hips back. Repeat 8 to 10 times.

Step 5

Repeat on the other side.

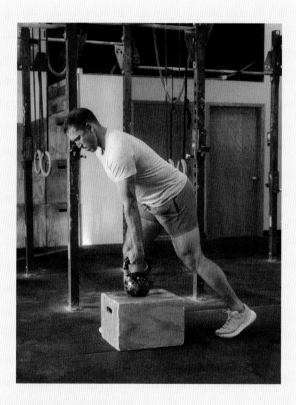

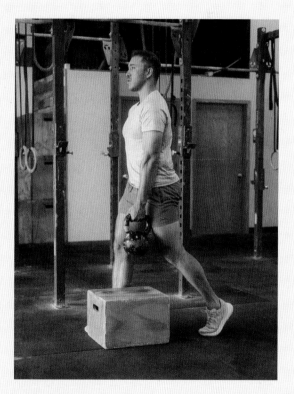

MODIFICATION 1

If less range of motion is more comfortable to start, place a prop underneath the weight.

MODIFICATION 2

If your lower back feels vulnerable as you hinge back and reach toward the ground, offload some stress by placing the bottom of your back foot on a wall and use it to support your body.

MOBILITY

Increasing mobility isn't always about the perfect exercise to isolate a joint. Sometimes, exposing the body to postures and positions that feel safe to perform while also challenging joint capacity is key. Maintaining healthy mobile joints can complement strength-building exercises, better preparing us for everyday activities like lifting suitcases into the trunk and picking up boxes in the garage.

And rather than avoiding movements that feel stiff or uncomfortable, there are benefits to safe exposure. Discomfort isn't inherently dangerous or bad; it could be a sign that a specific range of motion is underutilized or unprepared. Leaning into tolerable amounts of discomfort can improve overall mobility.

EXERCISES FOR MOBILITY

When improving mobility to pick things up off the ground, the main focus is the hips, ankles, and spine. The best strength exercises should challenge mobility and the best mobility exercises require strength. Remember, when training mobility, perform the reps slowly and explore as much active range of motion as possible. There is a big difference between "dumping into joints" and "actively exploring range of motion" of those joints. Dumping into a joint will feel forced, passive, and, potentially, pinch-y or uncomfortable. Actively exploring joint range of motion is slow and deliberate—it should feel challenging, not painful.

Where Should I Feel It?

These exercises target the hips, spine, ankles, and lower body muscles. The Gorilla Squat (page 101) challenges hip mobility and your upper back's ability to come out of a flexed-forward position. The ankle and knee joint range of motion is also tested with this movement, so you might feel the muscles in your lower leg and foot working as well.

EXERCISE 3

Gorilla Squat

For many people, the biggest barrier to lifting heavy things off the ground is having the strength and confidence to do so; for others, it's lacking joint mobility to squat down to the ground. The best way to improve your range of motion is to expose it safely to end ranges and build from there. The Gorilla Squat is powerful because it puts the lower body into triple flexion—hip flexion, knee flexion, and ankle dorsiflexion—while also challenging the spine in extension. Getting into a squat can be challenging because of pain, joint stiffness, or vulnerability, but incorporating a gradual exposure approach can be beneficial to building confidence and resilience in the lower body.

Step 1

Stand with feet slightly wider than shoulder-width apart, toes pointed slightly outward, between 15 and 45 degrees. Bend at the hips and reach your hands down to your toes and into in a forward-fold position. Place the backs of your hands on the floor so your fingertips are underneath your feet. Bend your knees slightly if needed. If you really struggle here, see the modifications (page 102).

Step 2

Keeping your fingertips underneath your feet, lower your body, bending at the hips and knees, dropping into a squat position. The goal is to get your hips below 90 degrees, dropping as deep into the squat as you can while maintaining an upright spinal position.

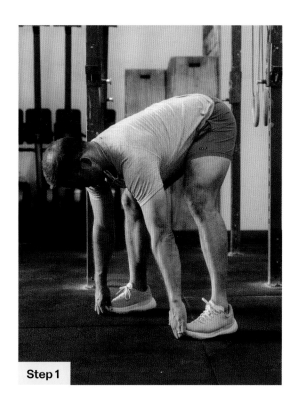

Step 1

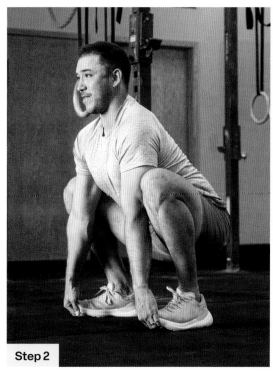

Step 2

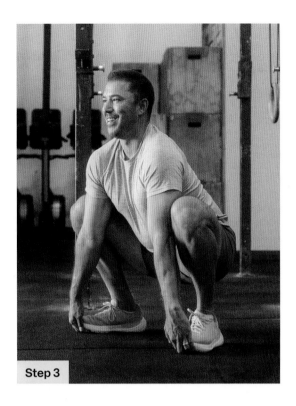

Step 3

MODIFICATIONS

If hip and lower back mobility are your main barrier, hold on to something like a door frame or a sturdy pole so you can sit your hips back farther and deeper into the squat. This will allow you to challenge the spine in a way that doesn't require as much hip mobility.

Also Try

The Deep Squat (page 40) will help you continue to build the mobility required in the hips, knees, and ankle joints to squat, stand from a seated position, and pick things up off the ground.

Step 3

In the squat, hold the position for 10 to 15 seconds, progressively pulling your chest through your shoulders to keep an upright spine, challenging joint mobility further.

Step 4

Come out of this position the same way you came into it: Pull your hips up out of the squat and into a forward-fold position, then return to a standing position. Repeat 4 to 6 times.

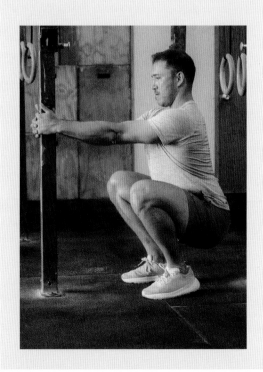

BALANCE AND CONTROL

Sometimes we lift things up off the floor with both feet planted in the same line, like with a squat or a deadlift. Other times, our feet are positioned one foot in front of the other in some variation of a split stance. Regardless, it is important to build lower body balance and control to prepare the hips, knees, and ankles for hinging and lifting.

EXERCISES FOR BALANCE AND CONTROL

Single-leg movements build confidence while balancing on one foot, which improves proprioception in the lower body. The hip hinge helps us evenly distribute our weight across our body while preparing to squat or reach for the floor. Well-controlled joints help the body work as one strong unit.

Where Should I Feel It?

In the balance and control exercises, you'll feel a lot in the entire lower body, primarily the muscles around the hip joint and foot. The Hip Airplane (page 104) works the glute muscles on the outside of the standing leg while challenging the small foot muscles. Similarly, the Standing Clamshell (page 106) works those intrinsic foot muscles of the standing leg. You will also feel this in the glute of the lifted leg.

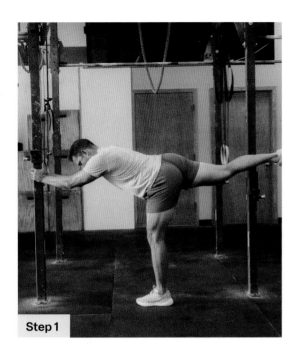

Step 1

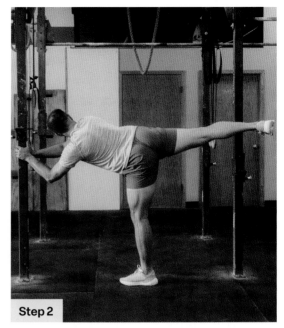

Step 2

EXERCISE 4

Hip Airplane

Of the many movements, exercises, and stretches out there, those that translate best to functional activities, like picking up things from the floor, mirror the demands on the body that the activity requires. The Hip Airplane not only challenges your balance, but also helps connect the hip muscles to the muscles in the foot gripping the floor—building control in the hip joint, connecting to the floor, and getting proprioceptive feedback from your foot, ankle, and all the way up the leg.

Step 1

Stand near a pole, a wall, or in a door frame with your body perpendicular to the wall the frame is in. Stand on one leg with your standing foot facing the door frame. Your standing leg's knee should be straight, but not locked out.

Step 2

Lift your other leg straight back behind you, close to parallel with the ground. Open the lifted leg away from the ground, stacking your pelvis over the standing leg.

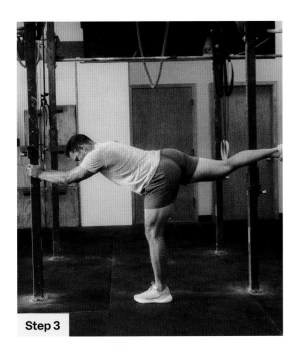

Step 3

If your balance is challenged, bend the floating leg at the knee to shorten the lever. This should allow for more movement control.

Step 3
With control, slowly roll the lifted leg back to where you started, with the front of your hips facing the ground. Repeat 6 to 8 times.

Step 4
Switch legs and repeat.

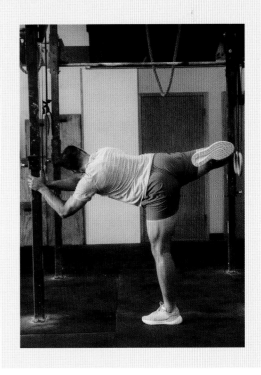

EXERCISE 5

Standing Clamshell

The standing clamshell is fundamental to building a base of support to lift from. With adequate control in the muscles, ligaments, and fascial slings of the posterior chain, we can more easily disperse force across the whole body. When this happens, the hips and supporting soft tissue can absorb force rather than the small joints in the spine.

Step 1

Start facing a wall, then step back 12 to 18 inches (30 to 45 cm) from it. With your hands on the wall, lift one foot off the ground, bending at the knee with your foot behind you.

Step 2

Lift the leg with the bent knee from the hip and out to the side as high as you can, rotating the pelvis over the standing leg. Hold at the top range of motion for 1 to 2 seconds.

Step 3

Bring the knee back to its original position. Repeat 8 to 10 times.

Step 4

Switch sides and repeat.

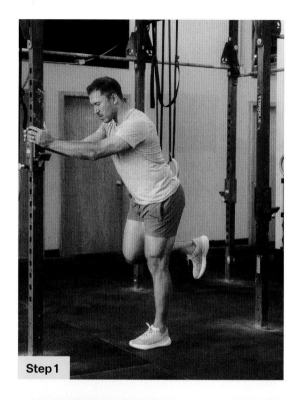

Step 1

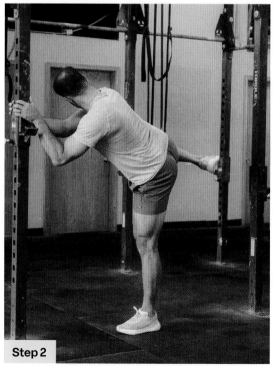

Step 2

MODIFICATIONS

The idea of rotating at the hips while balancing on one leg can feel unsettling. As you build trust in this movement, it can increase confidence in a more familiar range of motion. Instead of lifting the leg out to the side, drive that knee up toward the wall and then tap your foot back behind you while keeping your hands up against the wall.

CHECKING IN

Building strength while lifting things from the ground can be an ongoing practice. As you get comfortable lifting lighter items, lift heavier things. As you get better at lifting things from a raised surface, lift things from a lower surface. There are many variables you can adjust to challenge yourself. Continue to make notes, reassess, and find ways that continue to build trust in the body.

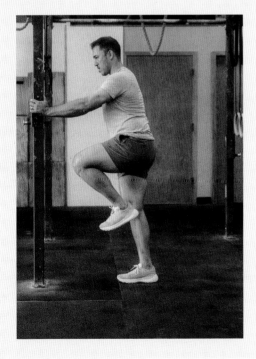

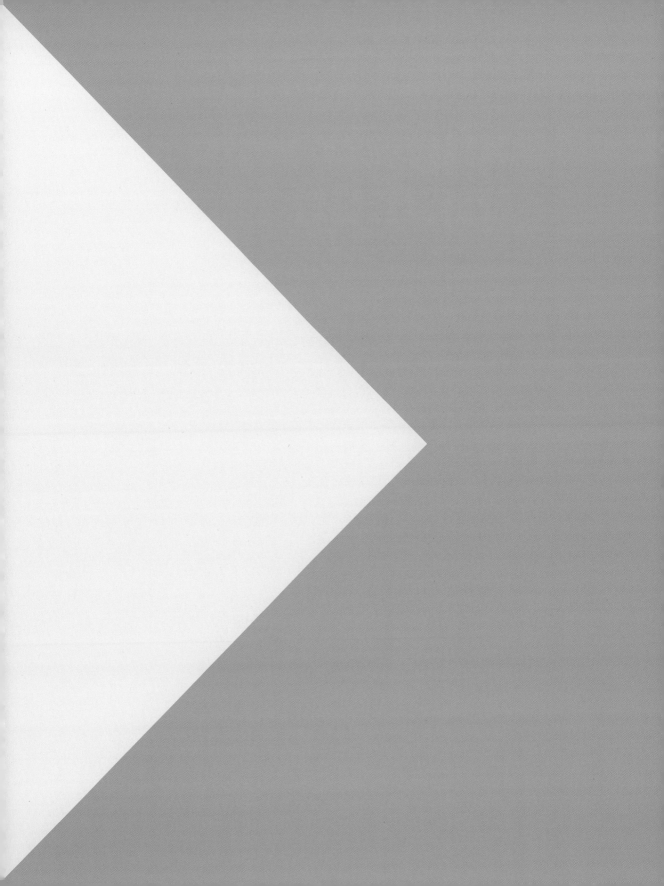

PART 3

Joint-Specific Movements

CHAPTER 10

FOOT, ANKLE, KNEE

The typical health care narrative often suggests we are fragile and must constantly work to "fix" our weaknesses, or "correct" imbalances. The truth, however, is that our body is remarkably strong and adaptable.

Increasing capacity in your ankles, feet, and knees is not about fixing something broken; it's about exposing your body to a variety of stimuli to increase the preparedness and strength of these key areas. These joints and their muscles are the foundation of our movement, supporting us in everything from walking, sprinting, and standing to jumping and climbing.

Our body is built to move and absorb force in many ways, but as we progress through life, there are many movements we do less frequently, such as explosive movements, single-leg balances, transitioning from side to side, bending or straightening the knee to full range—and so on. Finding ways to perform these activities in a safe way can keep us better prepared for what life throws at us.

These next chapters focus on individual body parts, not the whole system. The exercises are not a prerequisite for managing pain or optimizing strength or physical health. They are, however, valuable supplements with which to engage if you want to challenge these areas. You will cultivate a solid foundation that supports all your movements—from daily activities to athletic pursuits. You are not fragile; you are resilient, and with the right environment you can build the strength that allows you to move with confidence and freedom.

Try This: Knee-to-Wall Test

This a good assessment of ankle dorsiflexion, or your ability to bend your ankle, which is important in activities like walking, squatting, running, and jumping.

1. Place a measuring tape on the floor against the wall, perpendicular to the wall.
2. Stand facing the wall, one foot in front of the other, with the tested foot closest to the wall, toes of the tested foot touching the wall.

3. Drop down on to the back knee into a half-kneeling position for support.
4. Bend your front knee forward, attempting to touch the knee to the wall. Keep the heel of the tested foot flat on the ground.
5. If your knee touches the wall without the heel lifting, move the foot slightly away from the wall and repeat. Continue moving the foot farther from the wall, repeating the movement, until you reach the maximum distance where the knee can touch the wall without the heel lifting off the ground.
6. From your final position, measure and record the distance from your big toe to the wall.
7. Repeat on the other side and compare the distances. Some asymmetries are normal, but a significant difference is worth noting.

Interpreting the Results
- *Good dorsiflexion:* 4 to 5 inches (10 to 12 cm) from the wall
- *Limited dorsiflexion:* A distance significantly less than 4 inches (10 cm) could affect overall movement patterns and performance and is worth noting.

Note When you begin training for these knee-, ankle-, and foot-focused movements, it is perfectly acceptable to find different ways to support your body weight or modify the movements.

STRENGTH

Strong ankles, feet, and knees are crucial for maintaining overall mobility, stability, and function throughout life, allowing for more powerful and efficient movements. These joints and muscles bear the brunt of our daily activities. Strong knees absorb shock and distribute weight efficiently. Similarly, strong ankles provide stability and balance, preventing falls and sprains—especially important as we age. The feet, our foundation, support our body weight and enable movement; strengthening them can prevent common issues like plantar fasciitis. Focusing on these areas can improve overall physical resilience, reduce pain, and maintain independence and quality of life as we age.

Safety First Lower body strength movements require a lot of time under tension; using a prop for assistance can help.

EXERCISES FOR STRENGTH

The foot's anatomy is similar to the hand, however, we have far less dexterity and functional strength in the foot. These strength exercises focus on building that dexterity and control from the foot up to the hip joint.

Where Should I Feel It?

You will feel the strength-focused exercises that require balance in the arch of the foot and, potentially, all the way up to the hips. The Bulgarian Split Squats (page 115) challenge all the muscles in the lower body as well as the core. With the Knee Extensions (page 117), you will feel the top of the leg contracting in the quadriceps muscles and perhaps a stretch behind the knee.

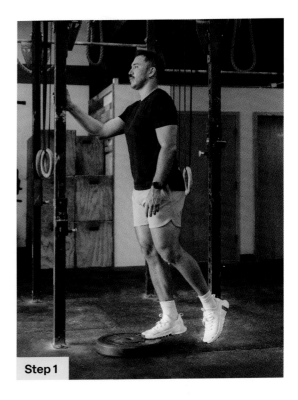

Step 1

EXERCISE 1

Balls of Your Toes Balance Work

Working on connecting through the balls of your feet can be an effective way to build strength, balance, and control throughout your foot and ankle. Being able to support yourself on one foot is a valuable skill for activities like climbing stairs, hiking, and putting on pants. The foot connects us to the earth and, for most activities, acts as our base of support. A simple ledge, stair, or a short prop, such as a book, can offer options to build strength through the foot and ankle.

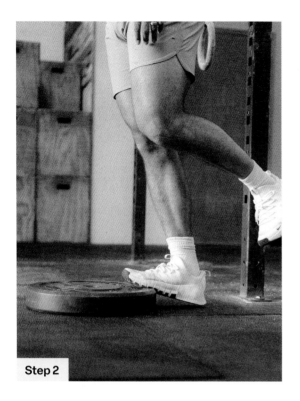

Step 2

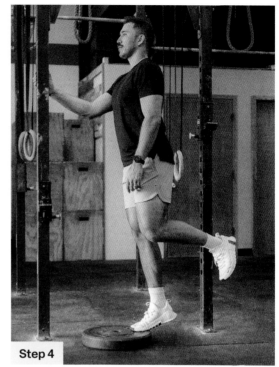

Step 4

Step 1

With one foot, step up on to your ledge, stair, or prop with the balls of your big toe and pinkie toe right at the front edge, your foot and heel hanging off the step. Your other foot can just float behind or to the side, as it is uninvolved.

Single Leg Balance

Step 2

Stand on one foot, as noted in step 1. Use a wall or a tabletop for support and lift your other leg. Unlock your standing leg knee so you are not using that joint to find balance. Equally distribute your weight across the ball of your standing foot and lift up onto your toes to root into the balance. Hold for 30 seconds (or your maximum hold).

Step 3

Repeat on the other side.

Calf Raise

Step 4

Begin in the position described in step 1. Drive up through the balls of your toes into a calf raise with one leg. You might tend to press more weight into the pinky side of your foot, so focus on equal weight distribution across the balls of your toes— from your pinky toe to your big toe. Lower to the starting position. Go slowly and complete 8 to 10 reps, then repeat on the other side.

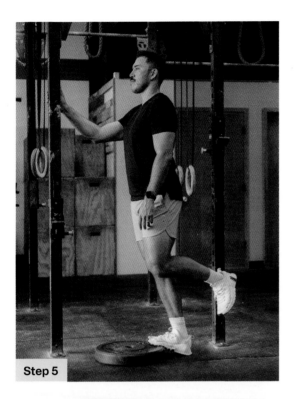

Step 5

Eccentric Calf Raise
Step 5

Begin in the position described in step 1. Drive up through the balls of your toes into a calf raise with one leg. Slowly pull the heel down, below the line of the prop, to find an active stretch in the calf. This cultivates range of motion in the ankle while actively loading the muscles around the joint. Each rep should take 5 seconds to drop down from the calf raise. Repeat 8 to 10 times. Switch to the other side.

Elevated Reverse Lunge
Step 6

A more advanced way to challenge foot and ankle strength is changing the way we load the foot from an elevated surface. Keeping equal weight across the balls of your right toes while standing on a ledge or prop, step the left foot back into a reverse lunge.

Step 7

Press through the ball of the front foot and drive the back knee up, out of the lunge and into a single leg knee drive at a 90-degree bend. Perform 4 to 6 reps (a full step back and then into a standing knee drive equals 1 rep). As you build strength and endurance, increase the rep count. Repeat on the other side.

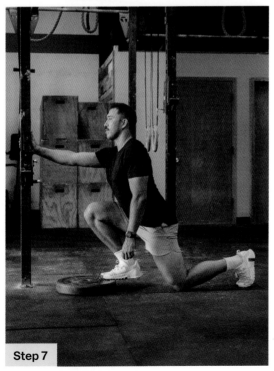

Step 7

MODIFICATIONS

Perform the exercises with both feet on the prop. If the Elevated Reverse Lunge (above) is too difficult for your balance, hold on to a prop or sturdy stick for support.

EXERCISE 2

Bulgarian Split Squats

Split squats build leg strength training and resilient knees. Having resilient knees lets us continue to climb, run, and jump as we age strong. Exposing the knees to controlled flexion and pressing off the ground into extension is a recipe for strong and able knees.

Step 1

Stand 2 to 3 feet (60 to 90 cm), or about a walking stride length, in front of a chair or bench. Extend your left leg back and place your left foot on the prop, standing strong and finding your balance on the standing (right) foot.

Step 2

Slowly lower the back (left) knee down toward the ground. Do this with an eccentric tempo, taking 3 to 5 seconds on the way down, or use a 1:1 tempo with a little more speed.

Step 3

Stand using the right leg for strength and the left leg for balance. Repeat this 8 to 10 times.

Step 4

Switch positions so the right foot is back on the chair and the left leg is your standing leg. Repeat.

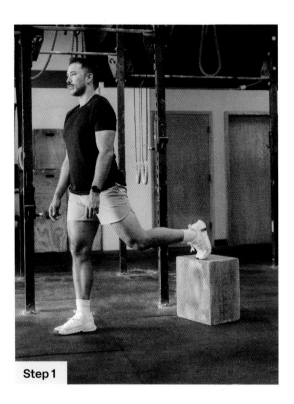

Step 1

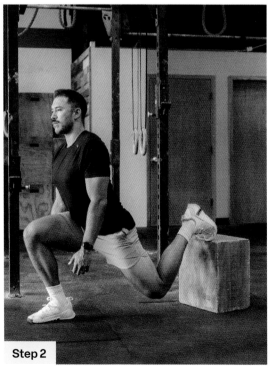

Step 2

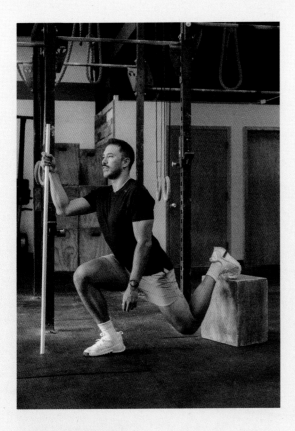

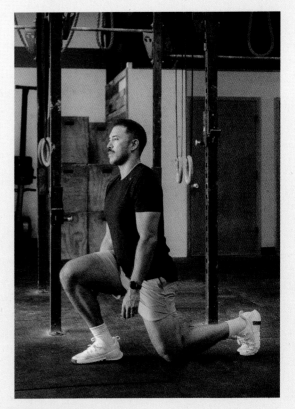

MODIFICATION 1

If balance is a challenge, use a broomstick or hold onto a countertop for support.

MODIFICATION 2

If keeping your back foot elevated is uncomfortable, lower the prop you have your foot on, or remove it and keep your back foot on the ground.

EXERCISE 3

Knee Extension

Moving the knee joint into extension safely can be helpful if the joint feels stiff or locked up. One simple way to do this is sitting and passively guiding your knee joint into extension.

Step 1

Sit on a chair or couch and put one foot up on a stool or bench, leg extended straight out, at about the same height. Make sure there is free space under your knee.

Step 2

Place the web of your thumb over your femur, just above the kneecap on your elevated leg. Guide your knee further into the straightened position (extension). Go slowly and listen to your body. Don't press through pain but explore some range of motion your knee may not have seen in a while. Remember, this is a very small range of motion. If everything feels good, complete 15 to 20 reps, slowly guiding the knee into extension.

Step 3

Repeat on the other side.

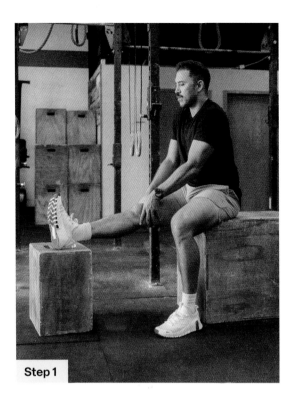

Step 1

MODIFICATIONS

There are many ways to get active knee extension. The knee extension machine at the gym adds resistance to straightening the leg. Walking uphill backward also exposes the knee to this range of motion in a more dynamic way.

MOBILITY

Unlike strength, which focuses on the power and stability of muscles and joints, mobility emphasizes the ability of these joints to move freely through their full range of motion. The joints here, though not big ball-and-socket joints like the hips or shoulders, can still benefit from building controlled range of motion. Fluid mobility in the knees ensures we can bend, squat, and move with ease, as well as adequately absorb force from daily activities like walking, running, and climbing stairs. Flexible ankles are crucial for maintaining balance and adapting to uneven walking surfaces, which can prevent falls and improve overall agility. The feet, which support our entire body weight, benefit from increased mobility to provide better shock absorption and distribution of pressure.

EXERCISES FOR MOBILITY

As with any active range drill, the more intention you put into it, the more you get out of it. Especially for the Ankle Circles (page 120) and the Tibial Torsion (page 122) exercises, it's easy to go through the motions. Focus on exploring as much range of motion as you can with every repetition.

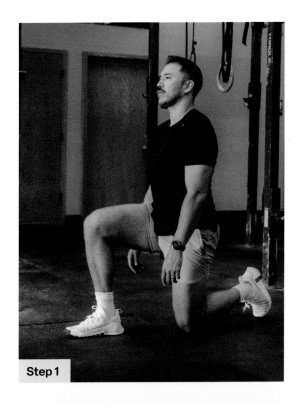

Step 1

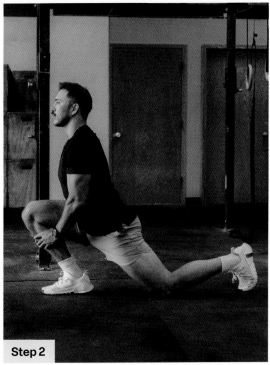

Step 2

Where Should I Feel It?

For these lower leg-, ankle-, and foot-focused mobility exercises, you'll challenge the supporting muscles such as the calf, the tissues around the shin, and into the plantar fascia at the bottom of the foot.

EXERCISE 4

Guided Ankle Dorsiflexion

Most often, we want to improve our ankles' range of motion for squatting down to the ground or getting up off a chair. The exercises from part 2 are your best friend to create more capacity for these daily activities. If you still want more, working through isolated movements to get the ankle in deep dorsiflexion can help you get the most out of your efforts.

Step 1

Get into a half-kneeling position (see Reverse Lunge with Reach, page 48), with one foot directly in front of you and the opposite knee on the ground.

Step 2

With both hands, grab your front leg just below the knee, with your fingertips overtop your shin and your thumbs on your calf muscle. Gently twist, or provide torsion to, your lower leg medially—if it's the *right leg, counterclockwise*; if it's the *left leg, clockwise*. The knee joint primarily flexes and extends, so this is a very small range of motion. Then, drive your knee over the middle of your foot to maximize ankle dorsiflexion. Don't worry if your heel comes off the ground; we want as much safe range of motion in this joint as possible.

Step 3

At the end of your range of motion, return to the starting position. Repeat 8 to 10 times on one leg.

Step 4

Switch your lead foot and repeat to work the other leg.

MODIFICATIONS

Instead of using your hands to provide torsion to the knee joint, place a weight, such as a kettlebell, on your knee and rock your weight forward over your ankle and foot. The knee will drive over the middle of your foot and then back to the starting position.

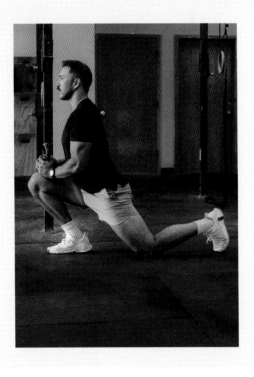

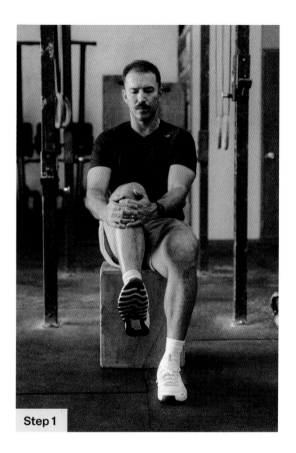

Step 1

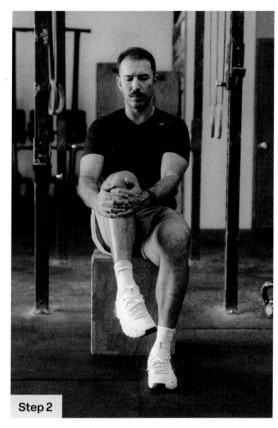

Step 2

EXERCISE 5

Ankle Circles

When working with the ankle, dorsiflexion isn't the only range of motion to build. Isolating controlled rotation in the ankle can free up range for activities like walking up stairs, running, and keeping balance. In this exercise, you will make a giant circle with the foot, isolating the movement to the ankle joint. Go slowly and explore the ankle joint's outer ranges—you'll see more control and improved range from the joint.

Step 1

Sit, or even lie, comfortably. Grab your lower right leg with both hands, with your fingertips over your shin to stabilize the tibia and fibula (the bones below the knee joint) to isolate the movement to the ankle joint.

Step 2

Bring your right ankle into maximal dorsiflexion— bring your toes up, rotate the bottom of the foot inward, and start creating that giant circle with your foot.

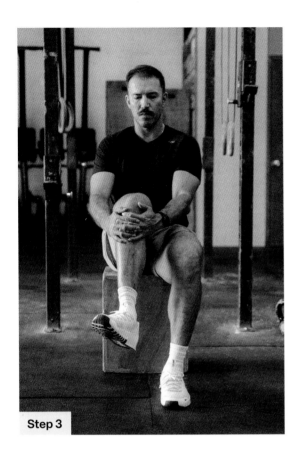

Step 3

MODIFICATIONS

Make smaller circles with your ankle, finding what works for you and your body.

Step 3

Continue through the range of motion: Point your toes down and finish rotating the bottom of the foot outward before pulling your toes back up to your shins to complete the circle.

Step 4

Continue with this range of motion, completing 4 to 6 circles in one direction, with each circle getting larger and taking up more space. Then, do 4 to 6 circles in the opposite direction.

Step 5

Repeat on the other side.

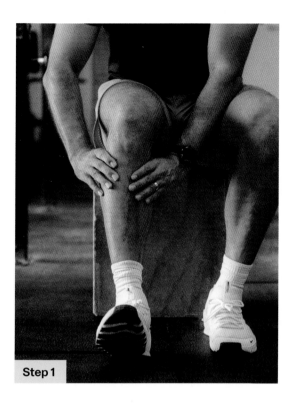

Step 1

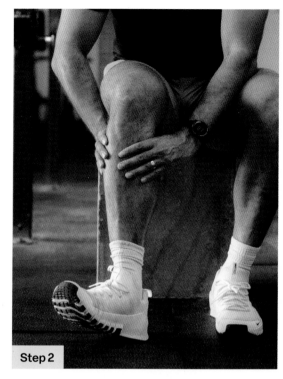

Step 2

EXERCISE 6

Tibial Torsion

Similar to Ankle Circles (page 120), we can also target mobility exercises to the knee. The knee joint is primarily a hinge joint, with its main range of motion being flexion, or bending, and extension. The knee joint craves stability and strength; however, training mobility in this joint can help with activities like squatting and climbing. In addition to flexion, though, the knee has another range of motion most people forget about: torsion, or rotation, of the tibia. This exercise will improve tibial torsion and could help unlock more depth in your squat or get rid of that knee pain when running.

Step 1

Sit on a chair, couch, or stool—something not too tall—and plant your feet firmly on the ground.

Step 2

Place both thumbs behind your right calf and your fingertips on the front of your right shin. Passively rotate your lower leg side to side without moving anything above your knee joint. Go slowly and avoid pushing through any pinching or pain. You don't need to force this; it's a very small range. If everything feels good, complete 6 to 8 reps (1 rep is moving to the right and then back to the left).

Step 3

Repeat on the other side.

MODIFICATIONS

Access this range of motion actively. Wrap both hands around your thigh (femur bone) with your thumbs on top and your fingertips underneath to generate movement at the tibia (the lower leg). Slowly rotate the lower right leg side to side. Complete 6 to 8 reps (one rep is moving to the right and back to the left). Repeat on the other side.

CHECKING IN

After working to increase your ankle, foot, and knee mobility, can you get down into a squat with more ease? Or is there less discomfort when you lift your leg to ties your shoes? I suggest revisiting part 2, specifically chapters 5 (page 30), 6 (page 46), and 8 (page 78), to see if you notice any changes. Remember, our bodies are diverse, and we all have our own timeline. Success is not always measured by assessments or tests. Sometimes, real success is recognizing the time and energy you are investing in yourself and your well-being.

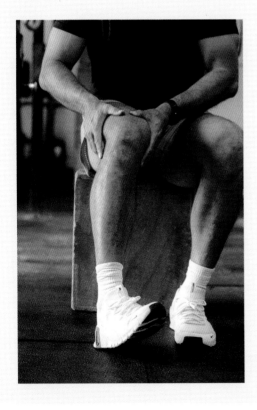

CHAPTER 11

HIP AND LOWER BACK

Sometimes, even when doing everything right, we can end up with tight hips or lower back pain.

This common reality usually involves two types of people: someone who gets frustrated, then avoids all movement and exercise, or someone overwhelmed with trying to understand their body who just powers through discomfort without making any changes.

There is a third approach, however, involving trial and error and self-awareness, that lets you explore what feels good and vary the stimuli you expose your body to. For example, if you do a lot of squatting movements and they don't feel great for your hips or lower back, try other activities or ranges of motion and revisit squatting movements later.

The hips and lower back are major players in many daily activities—whether picking things up off the ground, carrying items from point A to point B, or even getting out of our car. We require strength and mobility in these areas for almost everything we do!

Try This: Spinal Segmentation Test

Our spine is dynamic and can move in various ranges of motion; however, these ranges aren't challenged often. The Spinal Segmentation Test assesses spinal mobility. It evaluates the ability to control and isolate movement in each spinal segment, which identifies areas of stiffness or lack of mobility.

Note These movements can vary in difficulty depending on your current capacity. When working on hip mobility and strength, using props for support helps control how much body weight factors into the movement. It is important to find a movement variation that feels safe so you can build a strong foundation and progress.

1. Stand with your back against a wall, feet hip-width apart, 6 to 12 inches (15 to 30 cm) away from the wall, heels touching the floor. Your entire back, including your head, shoulders, and glutes, should touch the wall. Don't press your lower back into the wall. For this assessment, start in a position with a natural lumbar curve.
2. Slowly tuck your chin to your chest, initiating the movement from your cervical spine (neck).
3. One vertebra at a time, slowly peel your upper back away from the wall, moving from the cervical spine down to the thoracic spine (your upper back). Continue to roll down your spine slowly, feeling each segment move individually, until you reach the lower back—the last part to lift off the wall.
4. Reverse the movement, slowly pressing each vertebra against the wall—starting from your lower back, moving to your upper back, and, finally, your cervical spine. Work toward each segment of your spine contacting the wall, one at a time, in a controlled manner.
5. Perform the movement several times, paying attention to any "sticky" areas that feel stiff or difficult to isolate.

Assess

- Could you perform the assessment? Was there stiffness? Hesitation? Pain? If so, where?
- Did the movements feel smooth? Did you make modifications? (Step farther away from the wall; use your hands on your legs, etc.)

MODIFICATIONS

Place a small ball at the top of your spine for tactile feedback on your way down into flexion. However, this doesn't work when reversing the movement back up. If it's helpful, film yourself doing this assessment to add a visual feedback component to what you feel.

STRENGTH

The hips are the largest joints in the body, supported by some of the body's biggest muscles, including the gluteal muscles, hip flexors, and inner thigh muscles, which contribute to joint stability and movement. This area acts as the body's powerhouse, playing a vital role in nearly every movement we make. Strong hip muscles support and stabilize the pelvis, reducing the risk of injuries and improving balance and posture. Similarly, a strong, resilient lower back is essential for maintaining a healthy spine and supporting daily activities that involve bending, lifting, and twisting. Strengthening these areas helps distribute forces more evenly across the body, preventing strain and overuse injuries.

Safety First If you have an injury or medical condition—especially with the spine or the hips—consult your health care provider before undertaking these exercises.

EXERCISES FOR STRENGTH

Strength around this ball-and-socket hip joint is critical for activities such as climbing, jumping, running, squatting, and walking. Most exercises here highlight hip functions that are not as commonly used, such as rotation and lateral movement—varied stimuli that build capacity in the hip for the activities noted.

For the lower back, we will work on some deep core exercises, as well as challenge spinal end ranges of motion and segmentation—the ability to move each individual vertebra of the spine in a controlled and isolated manner rather than as a single unit. This skill is essential for maintaining overall spine health.

Where Should I Feel It?

These hip and lower-back strength exercises will be felt throughout the entire trunk. The Side Plank Clamshell (below) focuses on the oblique muscles and glutes. The Cross-Body Dead Bug (page 130) will be felt primarily in the deep core, especially while maintaining the neck and shoulder blades off the ground. The Hip Flexor Lift-Offs (page 132) will be felt in the front of the hip and into the quadriceps muscles of the leg.

EXERCISE 1

Side Plank Clamshell

The Side Plank Clamshell integrates both the glutes and the deep core and oblique muscles that support the hips and spine.

Step 1

Lie on your right side. Place your right elbow on the ground underneath your shoulder and your right knee on the ground with your other knee stacked on top. To start, your hips can be resting on the ground, keeping both knees bent with your feet behind you.

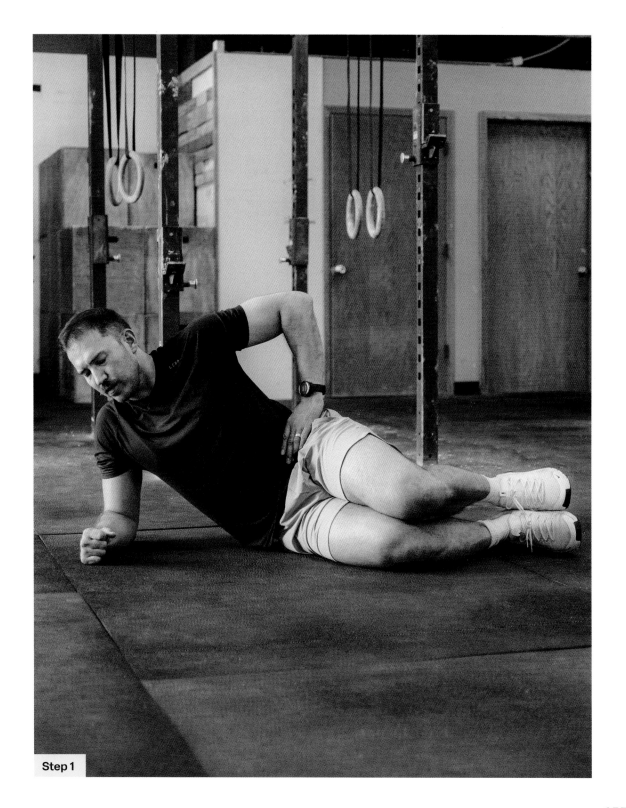

Step 1

Step 2

The first transition is up to a side plank from the elbow and knee: Drive tension into your elbow on the floor, lifting your hips off the ground. Knees remain bent, feet behind you.

Step 3

Come into a clamshell position: Keep your ankles and feet together and raise your top knee up and away from the knee anchored to the floor.

Step 4

Steps 1 through 3 are segmented so you understand how to perform the movement. Now, flow steps 1 through 3 seamlessly as 1 rep. Do 6 to 8 reps on the right side.

Step 5

Switch to the left side and repeat.

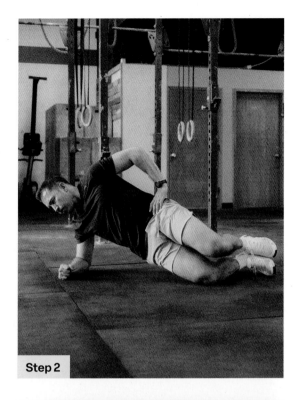

Step 2

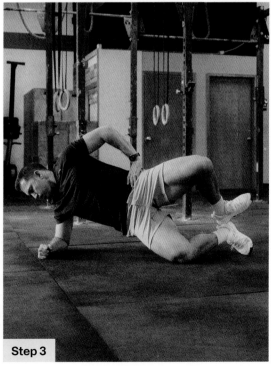

Step 3

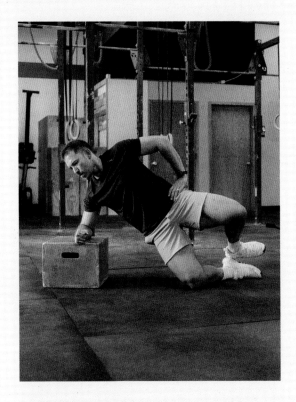

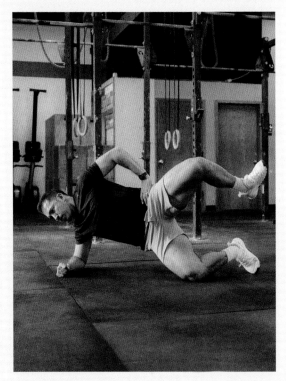

MODIFICATION 1

If this is too challenging for your core, increase the angle from the floor by placing a short box or prop underneath your elbow.

MODIFICATION 2

Turn this into an isometric exercise: Lift your hips off the ground and separate your knees while also lifting your top ankle, separating your feet. Hold your bent leg in this lifted position for 15 seconds (or your maximum hold). Repeat 4 to 6 times, then switch sides and repeat.

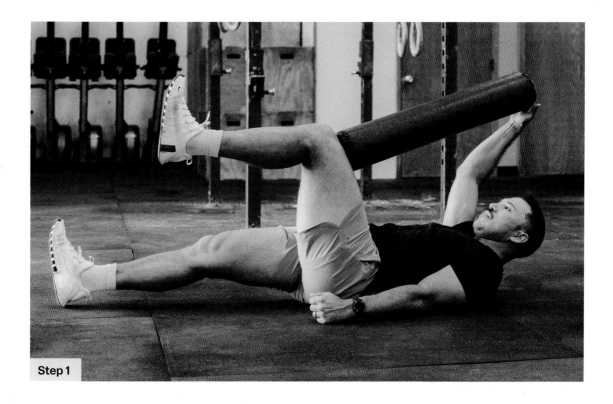

Step 1

EXERCISE 2

Cross-Body Dead Bug

This exercise is a full body integrator and a great primer before a workout, or to start your day. It prepares the core and hips for movements like rolling, getting up off the floor, and transitioning positions—all critical to maintain strength and independence with age.

Step 1

Lie on your back, bring your legs up to the sky, and bend your knees at 90 degrees so your knees are over your hips, shins parallel to the floor. Gently press your right hand into your left thigh above the knee to create a solid cross-body connection. If you have a short foam roller, yoga block, or prop, you can hold the prop and press it into the opposite thigh. Keep your shoulder blades and head slightly raised off the floor to challenge the core.

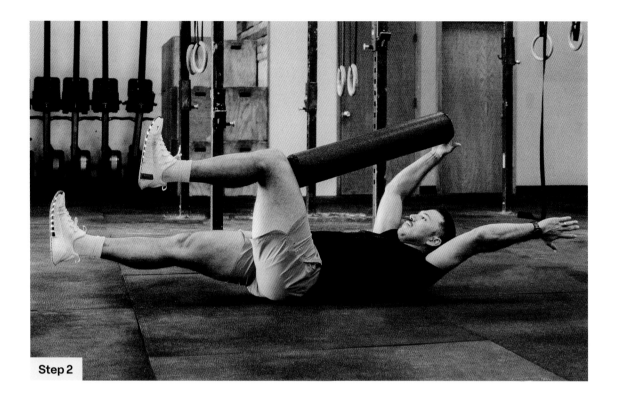

Step 2

Step 2

Draw your free arm and leg away from each other by reaching the left arm overhead and kicking the right leg straight while maintaining the cross-body connection established in step 1.

Step 3

Return the extended arm and leg to their starting positions. Repeat this movement 6 to 8 times.

Step 4

Switch sides and repeat with the other arm and leg.

MODIFICATIONS

Lie on your back, legs bent, feet on the ground. Alternate the legs in a marching movement. This gets the hip flexors used to this range of motion and provides challenge to the core as you lift one leg.

EXERCISE 3

Hip Flexor Lift-Off

Hip Flexor Lift-Offs challenge the front of the hip joint and build strength and control in the hip flexors, which are major players in movements such as standing from a seated position, lifting your legs to put on socks, or even climbing stairs. The hips flexors often get tight; finding ways to strengthen and build trust in movements that target these areas can help these muscles relax.

Step 1

Sit on the floor with your legs extended in front of you, your torso upright. Keep your toes flexed up, pointing to the ceiling. Place a small prop, like a yoga block, weight, or cup (anything from 3 to 6 inches [7.5 to 15 cm] tall to start), on the floor outside your right ankle.

Step 2

Lift your right leg up and over the prop to the ground. Most people tend to round their lower back to decrease the angle of the lift for the hip flexors. Keep your spine upright and your core strong to isolate the movement to the hip flexor as best you can. Lift the same leg up and over the prop, back to the starting position to complete a repetition. Complete the movement with as much control as possible, especially on the way to the ground after lifting up and over the prop. Repeat 6 to 8 times.

Step 3

Switch sides and repeat.

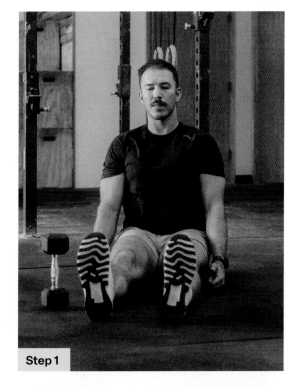

Step 1

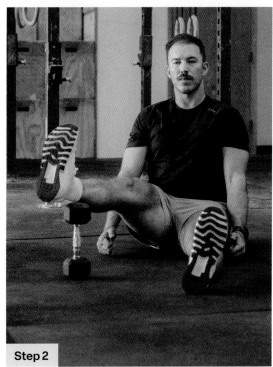

Step 2

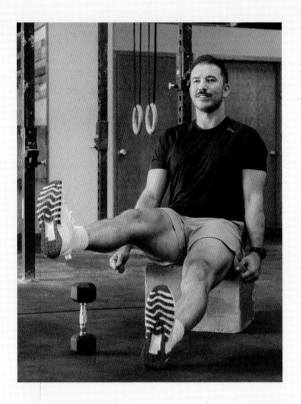

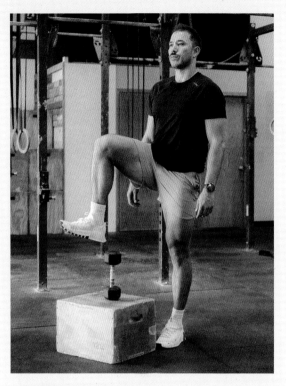

MODIFICATION 1

Sit on a prop or stool to decrease the angle and create less demand on the hip flexors while still working to keep your torso in a strong upright position.

MODIFICATION 2

Try a marching lift-off: Place your prop from step 1 on a box or bench in front of you. Place one foot on the box or bench next to your prop. Drive that knee up and lift your foot up and over the prop to the bench on the other side of the prop. This challenges the same muscles but makes the exercise easier if you have really tight hamstrings or tension in the backs of the legs when you straighten them.

MOBILITY

Strength is important for confidence in the hip and lower back, but mobility is important, too. The hips are pivotal joints that facilitate a range of motions, including walking, running, and bending. Limited hip mobility can lead to compensatory movements that strain other body parts, such as the knees and lower back. Similarly, the lower back needs to be flexible to support a variety of postures and positions, like bending to tie your shoes, swinging a pickleball racket with your friends, or lifting your kid when you get home. Without adequate mobility, the lower back can become stiff and deconditioned.

EXERCISES FOR MOBILITY

These mobility drills are not passive stretches; they are designed to be active. Move slowly and intentionally through the exercises, exploring as much pain-free range of motion as the joint offers.

Where Should I Feel It?

The 90/90 Transitions (below) and the Lateral Skater (page 138) challenge the muscles that support the hip joint, primarily the inner thigh and glute areas. The Cat-Cow Global Range (page 140) is felt more in the back and core muscles.

EXERCISE 4

90/90 Transitions

Many movements require the hips to move forward and backward, but rarely do we challenge these joints side to side or in rotation. This exercise exposes the hip joints to both internal and external rotation.

Step 1

Sit on the floor and place your legs in a 90/90, or Z, position.

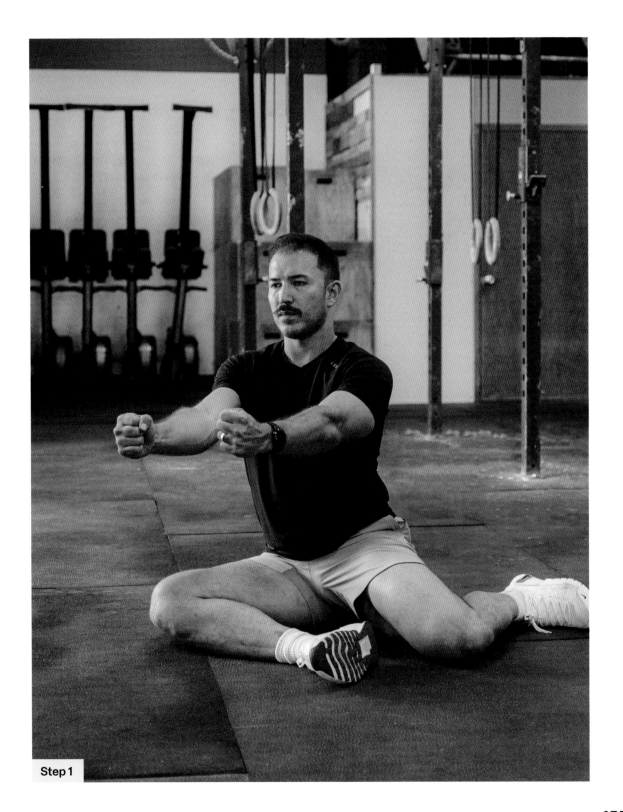

Step 1

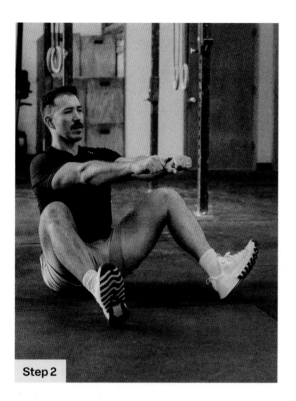

Step 2

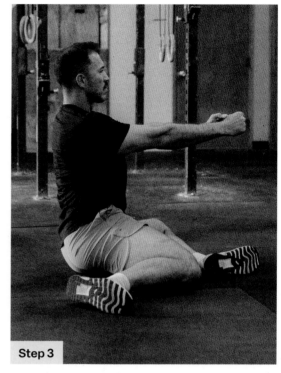

Step 3

Step 2

Create central tension through your core and your torso. While maintaining the same position with your heels on the floor, try to isolate as much of the movement as possible to the hip joints and begin to "windshield wiper" your legs to transition to the other side. Go slowly to focus on rotation in the hip joints.

Step 3

Transitioning to the other side, you will end up in the opposite *Z* formation. The leg that was formerly behind you in internal rotation will be in front of you in external hip rotation. Repeat this transition 6 to 8 times with control, isolating the hips as much as possible.

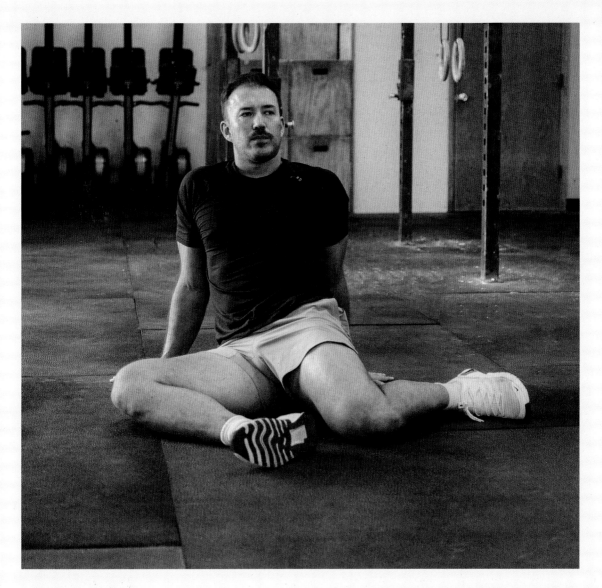

MODIFICATIONS

Sit on a short stool or prop, or lean back on your arms, to decrease the range of motion and the angle the hips need to rotate relative to your pelvis. As you work through this exercise, reduce the support from your arms to continue to condition the hip joints for rotation.

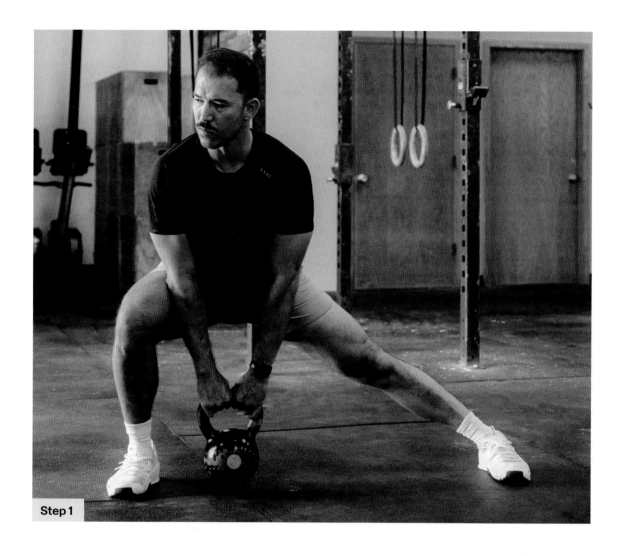

Step 1

EXERCISE 5

Lateral Skater

This exercise builds strength in a side-to-side capacity for the lower body. If you are just starting, you can do this exercise with just your body weight, but as you become more familiar with this range of motion, hold a prop or a weight while you do it for added challenge.

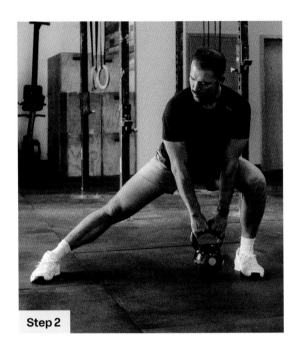

Step 2

MODIFICATIONS

If this creates too much stress on your knees, hips, or spine, use a table, chair, or countertop in front of you for support. As you build strength, rely less on the prop for support.

Step 1

If using just your body weight, keep your arms out in front of you; if you are holding a weight, choose something light to start and hold it with both hands, low between your feet, the entire time. Stand with your legs wide, about three times wider than hip-width apart. Your feet should be slightly pointed outward at an angle that feels natural for your stance. Hinge your hips back to one side and bend the knee on that same side, dropping your body into a side lunge.

Step 2

From this position, stay low and transition your weight to the other side, loading the other leg and ending in a side lunge on the other side. Stay low the entire time and transition side to side 10 to 12 times (5 to 6 times per side).

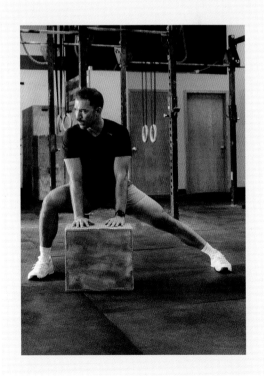

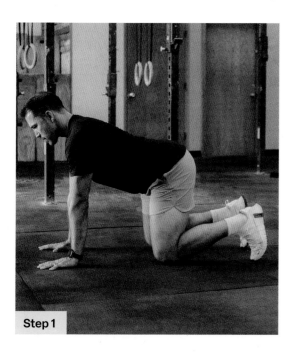

Step 1

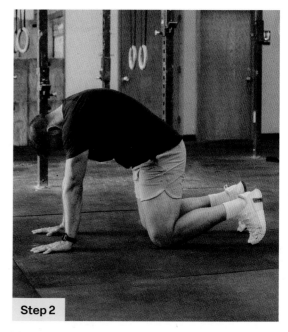

Step 2

EXERCISE 6

Cat-Cow Global Range

The Cat-Cow Global Range exercise exposes the entire spine to its full range of motion from a safe position. The goal is to find the end ranges of motion in extension (arched) and flexion (rounded) in both the thoracic (upper back) and lumbar (lower back) regions while providing a gentle, controlled stretch to some areas that might not typically move much.

Step 1

Position yourself on the floor in a quadruped position (on your hands and knees in a tabletop position), hands directly underneath your shoulders and knees directly underneath your hips. Keep your gaze down and pull your face gently away from the floor, creating a generally flat spine parallel to the ground.

Step 2

Come up into the cat position: Exhaling, round your entire spine toward the ceiling. Tuck your tailbone under, then sequentially round each vertebra in your upper and lower back. Allow your head to drop naturally, bringing your chin toward your chest without forcing it. Direct your gaze toward your thighs or navel. Imagine trying to create a smooth arch with your back, resembling a cat stretching its back.

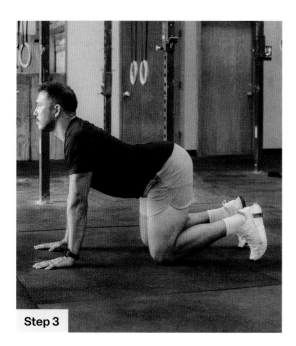
Step 3

Also Try

In this chapter, I introduce 90/90 Transitions (page 134), which challenge the hip joint during the transition between internal and external rotation, and focus on mobility in the hip joints, not specific to any particular movement or activity. To build mobility and capacity in the external hip rotators, required for getting up and down from the floor, revisit 90/90 Transitions with Grooving (page 56) in chapter 6, especially after spending time with 90/90 Transitions (page 134) to gauge any changes.

I also introduce the Cat-Cow Global Range exercise (page 140), which gets the spine into some end ranges of motion in a safe way. The Segmented Cat-Cow (page 90) from chapter 8 focuses more on moving each individual spinal segment with control. Having more spinal control helps when transporting or lifting heavy objects.

Step 3

Transition into the cow position: Inhaling, drop your lower back toward the floor, creating a gentle arch in your spine. As your spine arches, lift your head and chest toward the ceiling. Your gaze should follow naturally upward without straining your neck. Your spine should form a gentle arch. Your belly should drop toward the floor and your shoulder blades should draw together slightly.

MODIFICATIONS

If being in a kneeling position produces knee pain or discomfort, place some padding between your knees and the floor.

CHECKING IN

Building strength and mobility in the hips and lower back can take time. After working on these exercises for the next month or two, repeat the Spinal Segmentation Test (page 124). Do you notice any changes? Was the movement easier? Smoother? Working on these exercises can also support some of the movements and activities discussed in part 2, specifically in chapters 5 (page 30), 6 (page 46), 8 (page 78), and 9 (page 94). You are on your way to building a resilient body—keep it up!

CHAPTER 12

UPPER BACK AND RIB CAGE

As we age, maintaining upper back strength and mobility becomes increasingly crucial for preserving overall health and functionality.

The thoracic spine, or upper back, plays a pivotal role in ensuring endurance in certain postures and positions, as well as efficient breathing and functional movement.

There is no shortage of exercises for the neck and lower back on the internet, probably because a lot more people have lower back and neck pain than upper back pain. However, the upper back can be a great area of focus to support neighboring areas. By distributing loads more evenly across the spine, thoracic strength and mobility help the body work as a unit to prevent compensatory strains that can lead to pain and injury. It also enhances the ability to perform rotational and overhead movements, which are vital for daily activities like reaching overhead and participating in certain sports.

For those committed to aging stronger, performing exercises that enhance thoracic spine mobility and rib cage expansion can provide a sense of empowerment, improve athletic performance, and ensure a higher quality of life by maintaining independence and reducing the risk of falls.

Try This: Lateral Rib Cage Expansion Test

The ability to expand into your rib cage is an overall indicator of mobility in this area. This test evaluates the ability to engage in proper diaphragmatic breathing and utilize the rib cage for expansion.

1. Stand upright, or sit upright in a chair with good posture and feet flat on the floor. Wrap a soft measuring tape or piece of string around your lower rib cage, right below your sternum and where your rib cage splits. Cross it in front.
2. Take a deep breath in through your nose, focusing on expanding the rib cage laterally (out to the sides) rather than just lifting the chest or pushing the abdomen out. Observe the rib cage movement and note the measurement at the maximum expansion.
3. Exhale slowly and fully, knitting your rib cage in tight. Note this measurement.
4. Repeat this process for 3 breaths to get an average measurement.

Assess

- Observe the symmetry of the rib cage expansion. Both sides should expand close to equal.
- Note any areas of restriction or lack of movement.
- Document any areas of pain or discomfort while expanding or contracting through the rib cage.

Notable expansion of the rib cage during inhalation (depending on your size and other factors, at least a 1-inch [2.5-cm] increase) indicates good diaphragmatic breathing and rib cage mobility.

STRENGTH

Developing strength in the upper back and rib cage area is essential for many everyday activities. This area, in conjunction with the pelvis and the core muscles, makes up the body's trunk, where most power and force is generated for the hips and shoulders to do things like running, reaching overhead, throwing, lifting heavy objects, and so on. The muscles in these regions, including the rhomboids, trapezius, and intercostals, play key roles in maintaining strong, prepared postures, providing spinal support for lifting and carrying, and enabling efficient breathing.

EXERCISES FOR STRENGTH

Maintaining mobility in the spine is important. It is equally important to challenge the spine by bracing and resisting force. Incorporating strength exercises, such as those presented here, that build capacity for movement and loading in the upper back can lead to a more resilient body.

Where Should I Feel It?

These exercises challenge the trunk—you will feel it in your core and through the intercostal muscles between the ribs of the rib cage.

 Safety First While training these movements, think about "expansion." The rib cage expands with each breath, creating more room to decompress the joints of the spine and move the body. This decompression should create space and, with this, reduce feelings of pinching or compression. If you feel any of those sensations while practicing the movements in this chapter, slow down and focus on your breath. In the upper back and rib cage area, movements are small, so it doesn't take much to create change.

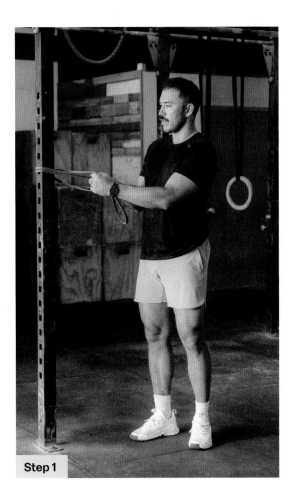

Step 1

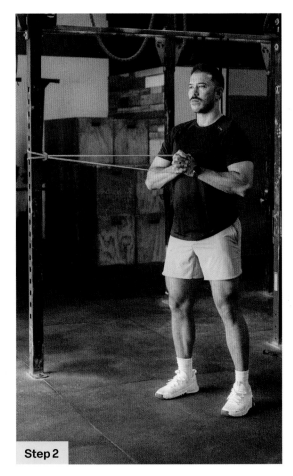

Step 2

EXERCISE 1

Pallof Press

This exercise has an anti-rotation focus and builds trunk strength by preparing our bodies to brace for sudden or unexpected force, like during a slip or fall. This exercise challenges your body's ability to fight against the lateral and rotational pull to the side and helps you with balance and core strength. You will need a long exercise band with light to moderate tension and something to anchor the band to a door frame or a squat rack.

Step 1

Loop the band around a door frame or a squat rack at about chest height. If you are setting this up on a squat rack or pole, loop the band around the upright structure; if you are putting it in a door frame, depending on how tight your frame is, loop it around the door handle on the other side of the door and pull the band through and close the door.

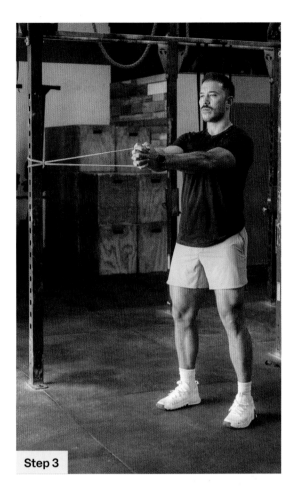

Step 3

Step 3

Recruit the muscles of your core, shoulders, and pelvis and press the band forward away from your chest, recognizing the lateral/rotational pull to the side but fighting to keep your body in an upright position through the movement. Hold the band out at the end of the range of motion for 1 second, elbows fully straightened in front of you, then pull the band back to your chest (the starting position).

Step 4

When you feel confident in this position and have your balance, perform 8 to 10 reps.

Step 5

Change your stance to face the other direction, switch your lead foot, and repeat on the other side.

Step 2

Stand in a split stance in a walking stride with your feet about hip-width apart. The foot closest to where the band is anchored should be the foot stepped back in the stance. Clasp your hands together around the band and hold the band at your chest directly in front of you. There should be significant tension on the band, but not so much that you feel like you are being pulled over.

MODIFICATIONS

Doing this exercise from a tall kneeling position with both knees on the ground, hip-width apart, can provide a stronger base of support. Slide the band down to chest height from a tall kneeling position and complete steps 3 through 5.

EXERCISE 2

Banded Expansive Breath

There is no single correct way to breathe. There are different types of breathing for different conditions, different capacities, and different goals. This exercise is not meant to teach you about all the physiological types of breathing and the reasons you might pursue them, but rather to show you one way you can use your breath with a biomechanical intent.

Most of us inhale either with our chest or through our belly, but 360-degree expansive rib cage breathing is less common. Expansive movement in the rib cage doesn't happen often and one of the only ways to do that is to use your breath to explore it. Just like a bench press or squat, this style of breathing is an exercise—not something to perform all day every day.

Imagine a balloon at the bottom of your rib cage that is being blown up and expanding in every direction. This can be challenging to achieve without feedback, so I really like this banded expansive breath exercise to find the associated sensation.

This core principle is from Foundation Training's Decompression Breathing techniques and has been one of the most powerful tools that I have learned when working with patients in pain or looking to build strength.

Step 1
Stand tall, grab a mini loop band, and place it around your lower rib cage.

Step 2
Familiarize yourself with the subtle compressive force around your rib cage from the mini loop band and inhale an expansive breath into the pressure while maintaining a tall strong posture, followed by an exhale, doing your best to maintain outward pressure against the band pressing around your rib cage.

Step 3
Take 6 to 8 breaths in and out using the band, 3 to 4 times throughout the day.

MODIFICATIONS

If you don't have a band, use your hands. Take both hands and cup the web of your thumbs around the lateral aspects of the rib cage as low down as you can. Avoid shrugging your shoulders up in this position. Complete steps 1 through 3.

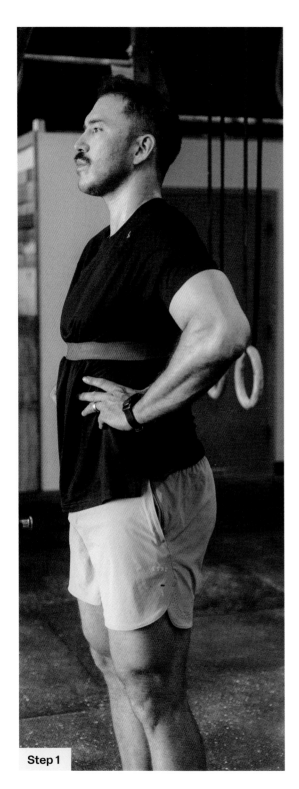

Step 1

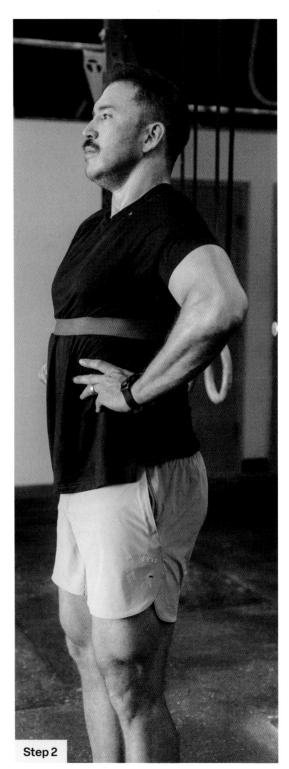

Step 2

MOBILITY

The upper back and rib cage range of motion is typically not challenged during daily activities—especially if you are sedentary for your job or spend a lot of time sitting, working on a laptop or device. As a result, your upper back stays stuck in flexion most of the day. The good news is that our body is built to withstand tons of force, but continuing to stay mobile and exposing our body to a variety of postures and positions builds a resilient body prepared to be challenged.

EXERCISES FOR MOBILITY

These exercises offer different ways to explore end range of motion in the upper back and rib cage by building rotation and extension in the thoracic spine.

Where Should I Feel It?

These exercises focus on the upper back area—and that is exactly where you will feel them. With the rotation and extension, especially, you may feel pressure in the spine. If it gets pinch-y or painful, don't push through it—back off the range of motion a bit until the sensation subsides.

EXERCISE 3

Kneeling Medicine Ball Circles

When working on building controlled mobility in the spine, the concept of irradiation comes into play. The area we are focusing on can relax when we build tension in surrounding areas. For example, holding something to create central tension throughout the core during the exercise allows you more capacity to relax and find more intentional mobility directly at the spine. If you do not have a medicine ball, grab a different prop, like a backpack, rolled-up blanket, pillow, or even a pile of laundry.

Step 1

Get into a tall kneeling (both knees) position, hip-width apart, and grab the medicine ball or prop. Wrap your arms around it and hold it tightly to your chest.

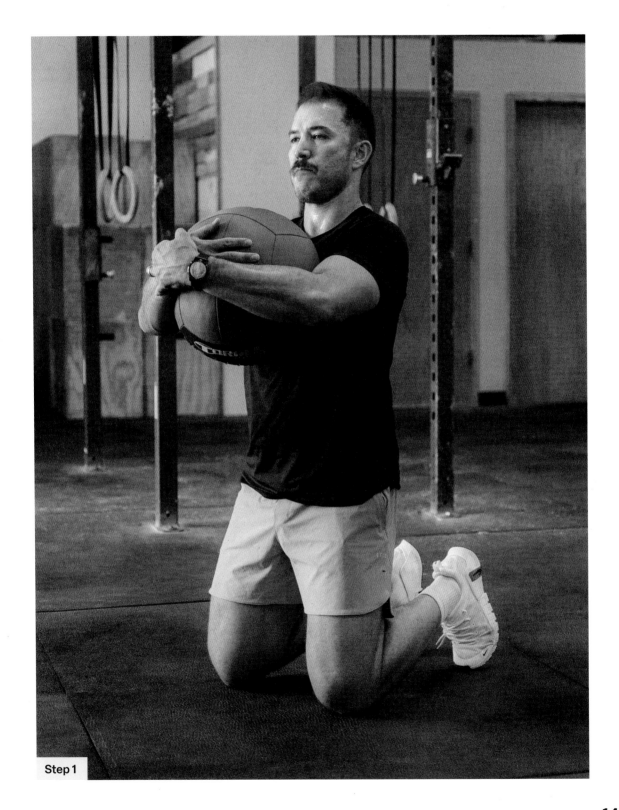

Step 1

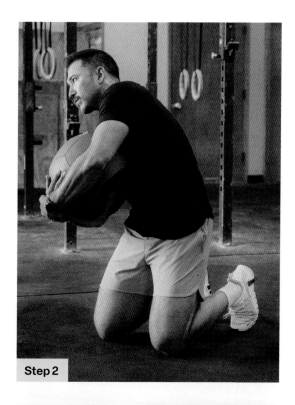

Step 2

Step 2

Mentally pinpoint a spot in the upper back between the shoulder blades and use that as the fulcrum of movement in the spine. Starting at the top, with your upper back bent back and your elbows pointed slightly up, begin to drop your elbows (and the prop) into a clockwise range of motion—in this case, starting to drop down and to the left. Focus on going slowly, with control.

Step 3

Continue making the giant circle, taking up as much rotation in the spine as possible until you get to the bottom of the range (six o'clock). At this point, continue to rotate back up to your starting point.

Step 4

Repeat 4 to 6 times in a clockwise direction.

Step 5

Repeat, making counterclockwise circles.

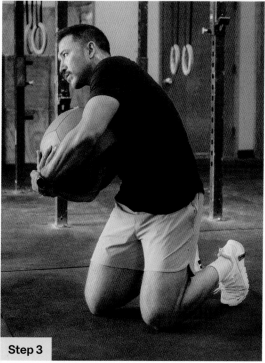

Step 3

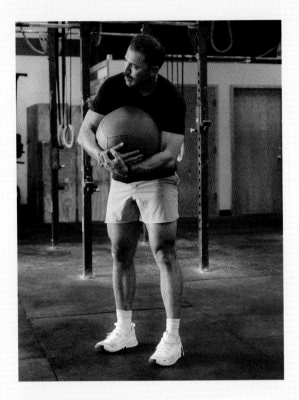

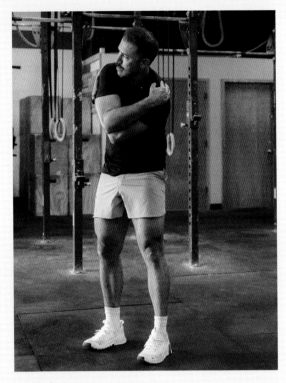

MODIFICATION 1

If kneeling is uncomfortable, perform this exercise in a standing position. Kneeling is preferred because it takes the legs out of the equation, leaving less room for the body to generate movement from other areas to complete the exercise, like the hips or even the knees.

MODIFICATION 2

You can also do this exercise without a prop by crossing your arms over each other, grabbing your shoulders to create the central tension, and rotating your elbows in a circle.

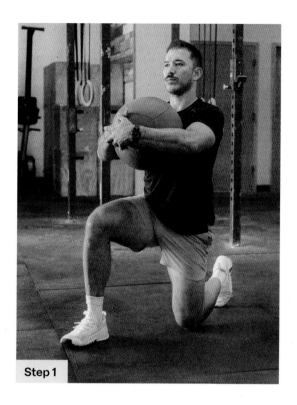

Step 1

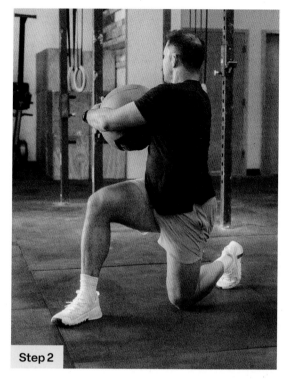

Step 2

EXERCISE 4

Half-Kneeling Medicine Ball Rotations

Similar to Kneeling Medicine Ball Circles (page 148), creating movement off a solid base isolates mobility to specific joints. In the half-kneeling position, there is an opportunity to build tension through the hips and legs and leverage more movement through the upper back. Restoring rotation through the upper back and rib cage means the body can move more easily, dispersing force during activity to a broader area of the spine so it's not only using the lower back to rotate.

Step 1

Drop down to the left knee and step your right foot forward into a half-kneeling position. Grab your medicine ball or prop and create tension off it by squeezing the ball tightly.

Step 2

Build a stable base in the lower body by holding strong and still through the legs and pelvis. Initiate rotation through your upper back as far as you can to the right without losing your lower body positioning. After hitting the end range of motion, return to center where you started. Repeat this rotation 6 to 8 times, staying tall the entire time.

Step 3

Switch your lead foot and place your right knee on the ground. Repeat the rotation in the other direction.

MODIFICATIONS

If you experience pain when on your knee, place a pad or pillow under it for support.

CHECKING IN

Layering in exercises from this chapter can also change how you feel during some of the activities in part 2, specifically in chapters 6 (page 46), 7 (page 64), and 8 (page 78). Work through this chapter for a few weeks and then retest the Lateral Rib Cage Expansion Test (page 142) to gauge any changes. Investing in your upper back mobility, rib cage expansion, and trunk stability plays a big role in maintaining a strong and independent body.

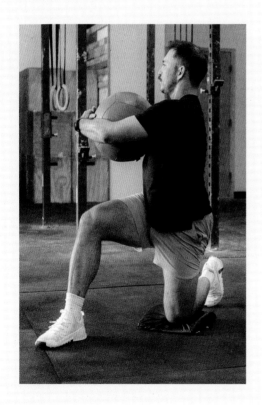

CHAPTER 13

SHOULDERS AND NECK

When talking about posture, a common thing I hear is, "Chin up! Shoulders down and back!" Although spending too much time with your shoulders slouched forward might not be great, neither is hyper fixating on pinching your shoulder blades together.

Posture is less about finding a "perfect" position to maintain and more about building endurance in muscles and exposing joints to their full capacity regularly so your body feels prepared for the wide variety of postures and positions you put it in.

The average human today spends the majority of time in one position: neck protruding forward, head heavy in front of the body, shoulders slouched anteriorly (to the front). I am a firm believer that this posture and position are not inherently bad; however, being in *any* isolated position for too long without exploring the full range of a joint's motion is less than optimal. The body craves movement.

Try This: Wall Angel Test

1. Sit on the floor with your back up against a wall, legs out straight in front of you. Ensure that the base of your spine at your belt line, upper back, and head are in contact with the wall.
2. Raise your arms to form a 90-degree angle at the elbows, with your upper arms parallel to the floor and your forearms pointing straight up, resembling a goalpost. Your elbows, forearms, and the back of your hands should also be in contact with the wall.
3. Slide your arms up the wall, maintaining contact with the wall with all of the areas noted in step 2 until your arms are fully extended overhead, forming a *Y* shape.
4. Reverse the movement, sliding your arms back down to the starting position. Perform the movements slowly and with control.

Assess

- Could you keep contact with the wall throughout the movement, particularly the lower back, upper back, head, elbows, and hands? If not, how far up were you able to get while maintaining contact?
- Was the reach overhead symmetrical? Asymmetries are normal in the human body, but they are still good to note.
- Was there any pain or discomfort during the movement? If so, this may need further assessment or intervention.

STRENGTH

The neck and shoulders are involved in almost every movement of the upper body, providing support and mobility for the head, arms, and torso. The pain experience, as we discuss in part 1 (page 10), is diverse and many factors contribute to it. Building strength in your neck and shoulders will not guarantee that you will never have a neck or shoulder injury. That said, strong neck and shoulder muscles stabilize the cervical spine, better preparing our bodies for reducing the risk of strains and sprains, which are common because of extended times in certain postures or sudden, unexpected movements.

 Safety First If you experience any neck pain, do not push through it. As always, if something doesn't feel right, consult your health care provider.

EXERCISES FOR STRENGTH

Strength training for the shoulder muscles, including the deltoids, rotator cuff, and trapezius, contribute to the shoulder joint's stability and motor control, which is crucial for a range of activities—from lifting and carrying to pushing and pulling. Some of these exercises explore big ranges of motion in joints that may not get a ton of movement throughout the day. Depending on your current capacity, you may experience stiffness or even discomfort. If this happens, back off the range of motion and see if your tolerance to the movement starts to grow.

Where Should I Feel It?

You will feel the neck isometrics in the small stabilizing muscles of the spine and maybe even the shoulders. For the Prone Shoulder Lift-Off (page 158), expect to feel it through the back of the shoulders. The Scapular Push-Ups (page 160) target the serratus muscles (along the side of the rib cage and the shoulder blade) and rhomboids (between the shoulder blades).

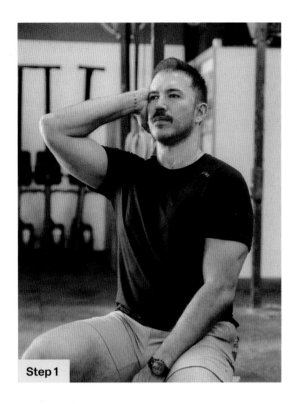

Step 1

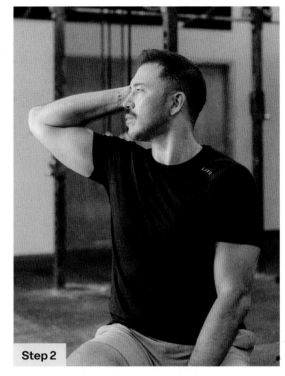

Step 2

EXERCISE 1

Hand-Resisted Neck Isometrics

This drill builds endurance in the small spinal stabilizing muscles of the neck and increases rotation and lateral flexion in the neck, ranges of motion important for activities like shoulder-checking while driving or turning to talk to someone next to you.

Step 1

Sit or stand in a comfortable position. Raise your right hand and place your right palm next to your cheekbone. Begin to generate force from the neck into your hand, creating an isometric contraction into your palm. Hold this contraction for 7 to 10 seconds. Repeat 3 times.

Step 2

Rotate your neck to the right side as far as you comfortably can. Place your right palm on your right cheek and repeat step 1. If you feel stiff and your range of motion feels limited, do this in your comfortable range, but after completing the hold, retest your range of motion to see if there's any improvement. If yes, repeat the next reps in your new range. If no, repeat the exercise in the original range of motion in the first part of this step.

Step 3

Starting back at center in an upright position, bring your right palm to your forehead. Once again, generate force from the neck into your hand, creating that same isometric contraction into your palm. Hold this contraction for 7 to 10 seconds. Repeat 3 times.

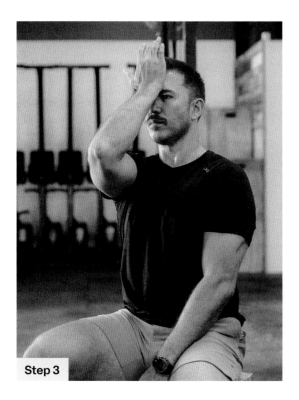

Step 3

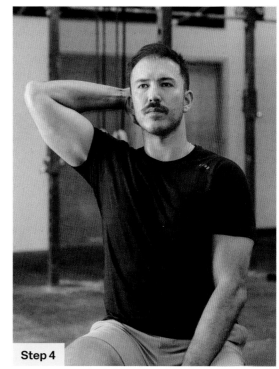

Step 4

Step 4

Return to the original upright position (step 1). This time, bring your right hand behind your head and build force from the neck into your hand. Hold this isometric contraction for 7 to 10 seconds. Repeat 3 times.

Step 5

Repeat steps 1 through 4 with your left hand, on your left side.

MODIFICATIONS

The neck can be vulnerable. To decrease this vulnerability, apply less pressure from the hand or create more support for the head during the exercise, such as by sitting in a chair against a wall and resting the back of your head against the wall.

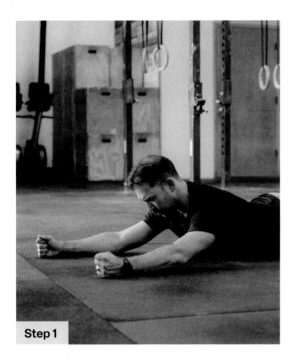

Step 1

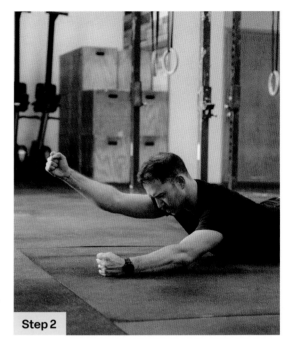

Step 2

EXERCISE 2

Prone Shoulder Lift-Off

As discussed in chapter 7 (page 64), reaching overhead is a critical skill to maintain while aging strong. Prone Shoulder Lift-Offs can support this activity, building strength in the shoulders and the deep neck flexor musculature.

Step 1

Lie flat on the floor, facedown, with your arms reaching overhead in a *Y* shape. Make two fists and place the pinkie sides of your hands on the floor with your thumbs pointed up to the ceiling. Gently pull your face away from the ground, maintaining length in the back of the spine and working the small muscles in the front of the neck.

Step 2

Lift one fist 1 to 2 inches (2.5 to 5 cm) off the ground while maintaining control and stillness in the rest of the body. You might feel additional pressure drive into the fist that remains on the ground—that's okay, as long as you maintain the integrity of the neck position and keep your face pulled away from the floor. Do not arch your lower back to achieve the range of motion in your shoulders.

Step 3

Hold at the top of this range of motion for 2 to 3 seconds. Repeat 4 to 6 times.

Step 4

Repeat on the other side.

MODIFICATIONS

Doing this exercise lying prone on the floor can be challenging. You can do it kneeling on the floor in front of a bench, chair, or couch with your arms on the prop in front of you, or standing against a wall with your arms reached up overhead against the wall. With either modification, maintain the same mechanics as the original exercise: face pulled away from the space in front of you to challenge the deep neck flexor muscles and isolate the movement to the shoulders. Avoid arching your spine to achieve the shoulder range of motion.

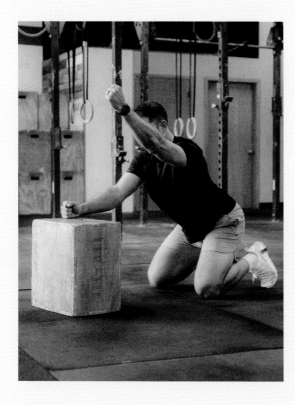
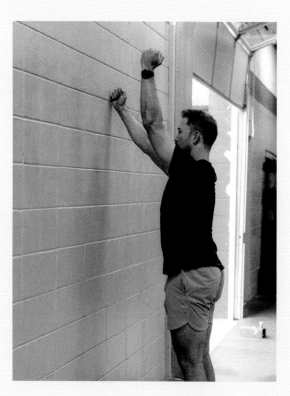

EXERCISE 3

Scapular Push-Ups

This chapter focuses a lot on the ball-and-socket shoulder joint, but another important relationship in the shoulder girdle is between the shoulder blade (scapula) and the rib cage. Scapular Push-Ups build strength and control in this area.

Step 1

Start in a plank position: hands under your shoulders, feet hip-width apart with your toes on the ground, your body in a straight line. Keeping your elbows straight, lower your chest toward the floor by pulling your shoulder blades together, retracting them over your rib cage.

Step 2

Push your chest away from the floor by spreading your shoulder blades apart, protracting them over your rib cage without bending the elbows at all. The arms stay straight throughout this exercise, isolating the movement to the shoulder blade area.

Step 3

Steps 1 and 2 combined equals 1 rep; do 8 to 10 reps.

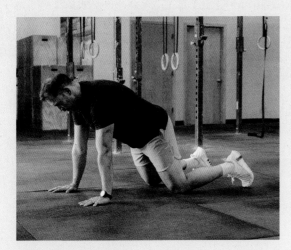

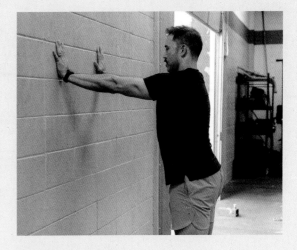

MODIFICATION 1

Do this in a tabletop position, with your hands and knees on the ground. This eliminates the lower body as a variable for movement and can help isolate the movement to the scapula without so much demand from the core muscles.

MODIFICATION 2

You can also perform this exercise from a wall. Stand arm-distance away from a wall and place both hands on the wall at about shoulder height. Repeat the steps as if you were in plank position on the floor.

MOBILITY

Whether you're reaching for items on a high shelf, lifting and carrying luggage, or putting on a jacket, flexible shoulders facilitate these movements smoothly and efficiently. Maintaining mobility in your neck and shoulders is important for performing daily tasks with ease and without discomfort.

EXERCISES FOR MOBILITY

These mobility exercises explore pain-free range of motion. It is important to expand these ranges in a safe way so you can do things like turn your neck to talk to someone sitting behind you, reach overhead to adjust the shower head, grab things out of the car's backseat, and put on your seatbelt.

Where Should I Feel It?

Neck Circles (page 162) will create a stretch along the neck muscles and the tops of the shoulders. You should feel the Lateral Shoulder Wall Crawl (page 164) and the Half-Kneeling Shoulder Wall Circles (page 165) in the muscles that support the shoulder girdle, as well as the joints in the upper back and the ball-and-socket of the shoulder.

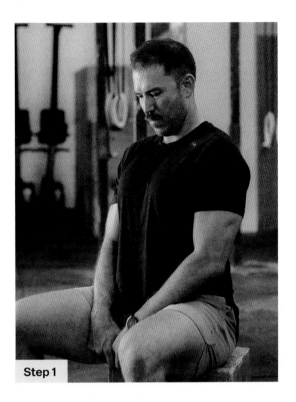

Step 1

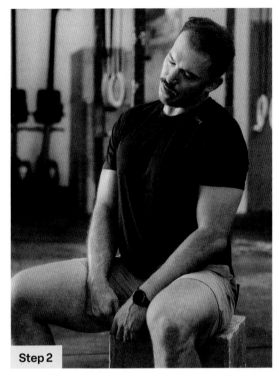

Step 2

EXERCISE 4

Neck Circles

The neck is uniquely configured to allow a range of movements, including flexion, extension, rotation, and lateral bending. We typically don't access all of this range of motion daily, so neck circles can be critical to maintaining mobility and improving neck health, alleviating stiffness, and reducing tension in the neck and upper shoulders, common areas where stress tends to accumulate.

Remember, when doing this movement (and any movement), do not push through any pain or pinching. If you experience any throughout the arc of this exercise, pause and find a narrower path that does not create resistance. Because of this, it is important to go slowly and explore your pain-free range of motion.

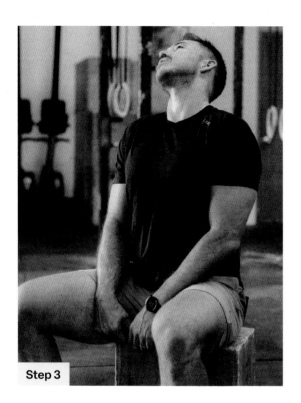

Step 3

Step 3

As you continue the rotation, when your chin is near your left shoulder, flex your left ear to your left shoulder and drop your head back (still drawing the circle with your chin, now pointed up to the ceiling), then work your way back down toward the other side to the starting position, completing your circle.

Step 4

From the starting position, repeat the circle 3 to 4 times to the left. Pay attention to the range of motion each time and make notes on what you observe.

Step 5

Repeat an equal number of circles, now to the right.

Step 1

Sit or stand in a comfortable position. Relax your shoulders and drop your chin down to your chest into full flexion.

Step 2

Roll your head to the left, drawing your chin toward your left shoulder, covering as much pain-free range of motion as you can. Think about drawing the largest circle you can with your chin.

EXERCISE 5

Lateral Shoulder Wall Crawl

This exercise is used as a rehab tool with patients who have rotator cuff injuries or frozen shoulder. For someone with healthy shoulders, it is an effective way to safely explore more range of motion in shoulder abduction—raising your arm out to the side—a motion that supports activities like lifting overhead or climbing/pulling from an overhead position.

Step 1

Stand sideways, parallel to a wall, 16 to 24 inches (40 to 60 cm) from the wall, feet facing forward. Reach your hand closest to the wall to the wall at shoulder height.

Step 2

Keeping your entire torso still, isolate the movement to the shoulder and slowly walk your fingers up the wall—your elbow will extend as your hand reaches overhead— until your arm is straight and your elbow is completely extended.

Step 3

Walk your hand back to the starting point. Repeat 8 to 10 times.

Step 4

Switch to the other side and repeat 8 to 10 times.

Also Try

You can also try the Forward Single-Arm Wall Walks (page 174) for a variation that tests shoulder flexion by facing the wall.

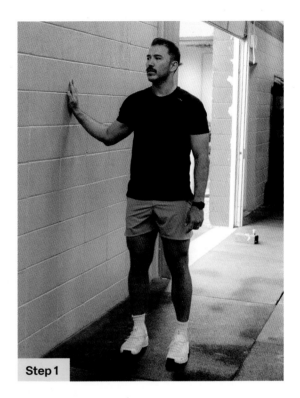

Step 1

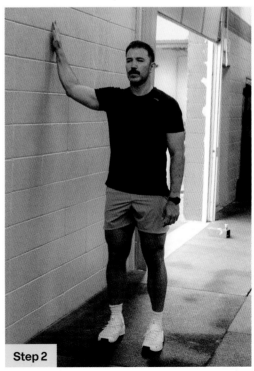

Step 2

MODIFICATIONS

If this feels challenging, stand farther, 18 to 30 inches (45 to 75 cm) from the wall, so when your elbow is fully extended, your hand isn't as far up the wall.

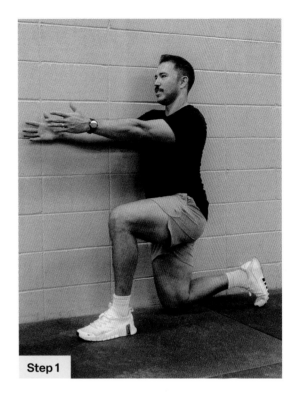

Step 1

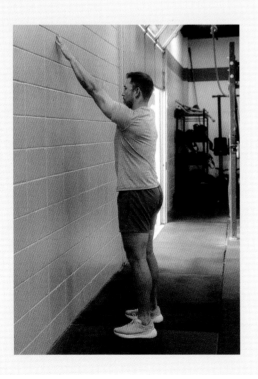

EXERCISE 6

Half-Kneeling Shoulder Wall Circles

These wall circles leverage the wall to challenge the mobility in your shoulder joints, as well as your upper back and lower neck area.

Step 1

Set yourself up against a wall in a half-kneeling position parallel to the wall. The leg closest to the wall is your lead foot, with your knee bent and foot on the ground; your other (outside) leg is bent, with your knee on the ground and foot behind you. Reach both arms out in front of you at about shoulder height, palms facing each other, parallel to the wall.

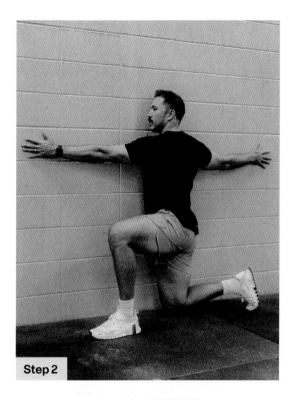

Step 2

Step 2

Flip the palm of the hand closest to the wall over to face the wall and place your fingertips on the wall. Begin to trace a giant half circle on the wall, allowing space for your head and neck to follow your hand.

Step 3

Continue the half circle down to the other side of the wall, following with your gaze, which is now behind you. When you reach the end of the range of motion, leverage pressure from your tracing hand into the wall to create more rotation and stretch through the shoulders and spine.

Step 4

Trace back to the starting position to complete 1 full rep. Repeat 6 to 8 times.

Step 5

Reposition your body, switch to the other side, and repeat.

CHECKING IN

It's always a good idea to give these movements time to progress. Making notes is a valuable way to reflect as you track your progress. Revisit part 2, specifically chapter 7 (page 64), and see how reaching overhead feels now that you've gained even more strength and mobility in these areas.

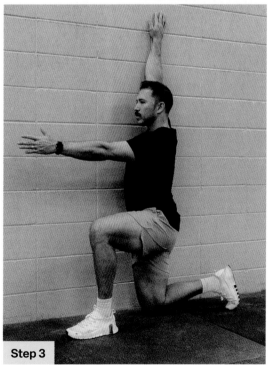

Step 3

ACKNOWLEDGMENTS

To my team at The Center of Movement: Josh, Justine, Julia, Andy, Bobby, Michael, and more, I'm grateful to link arms with you, to create with you, and to be in your circle of influence. You inspire me daily. I'm honored to work alongside you, pushing our vision forward, committing to empowering and educating people to make confident decisions about their health.

To Eric Goodman and the Foundation Training team: When I felt lost in this profession, the systems you created with Foundation Training and the way you communicated human movement and pain management provided the clarity I was looking for to better serve my patients in alignment with my values. I am forever grateful for the opportunities to work with the incredible team you have built. The connections I have made through the FT community are ones I will cherish forever. Thank you, Eric.

To my patients and community: Your trust in me is such a gift. From one-on-one patient care to community events, being in your presence and having the opportunity to work with you is what allows me space to learn and grow as a clinician and a human being. Thank you.

To my family: First and foremost, to my wife, Britny, for being my sounding board, driving so I could write, helping me get the ideas out of my head and onto paper, and forever being my support system with work, at home, and in life. To my parents, siblings, and in-laws, Rob, Marlene, Steph, Riley, Rylan, Jay, Nathan, Roni, Lacey, Cody, Aubrey, and Craig, for the feedback and encouragement, and supporting my commitment to this project over the last year. And last, but not least, to my daughters, Nara and Georgia, for the endless snuggles and curious questions: Love you two.

ABOUT THE AUTHOR

Dr. Matt Wiest is a Doctor of Chiropractic, pain management specialist, meditation and stress management coach, and founder/CEO of The Center of Movement, a group focused on educating and empowering people to discover sustainable solutions to support their physical, mental, and social wellbeing, and @dr.matt_tcom, which has over 1.5 million followers across Instagram, TikTok, and Facebook. Matt is also on the teaching staff of a global back pain and longevity company where he trains neurosurgeons, orthopedic surgeons, family physicians, physical therapists, chiropractors, and personal trainers from around the world. He has also been a keynote speaker for lululemon, Delta Airlines, and Four Seasons on the subjects of wellness and fitness. In his free time, Matt enjoys hockey, rugby, hiking, yoga, connecting with interesting people, hearing their stories, and spending time with his wife, Britny, and their daughters, Nara and Georgia.

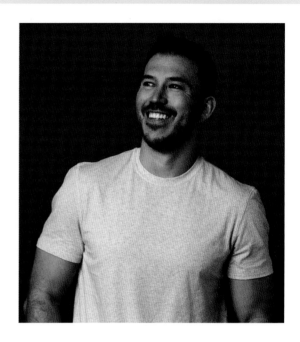

REFERENCES

Chapter 4
"Social Participation and Health: A Cross-Sectional Study Among Older Adults in Norway," published in *BMC Public Health*.

Smith, R., Segal, L., & McNally, S. (2009). *Disability weights for the Global Burden of Disease 2004 update: an analysis using Australian data.* PLOS Medicine, 6(11), e1000316. https://doi.org/10.1371/journal.pmed.1000316

Shin, J. Y., Kim, J. K., & Kim, J. (2018). *The relationships between physical activity, leisure-time activity, and academic stress in Korean adolescents: a cross-sectional study.* BMC Public Health, 18,907. https://doi.org/10.1186/s12889-017-4308-6

INDEX